The
MATRIλ
Principle

By R. S. Laura
& K. R. Dutton

John Magee Inc.
65 Broad St., Boston, Mass. 02109
Tel 617-695-9292 • 800-822-3007
Fax 617-695-1436

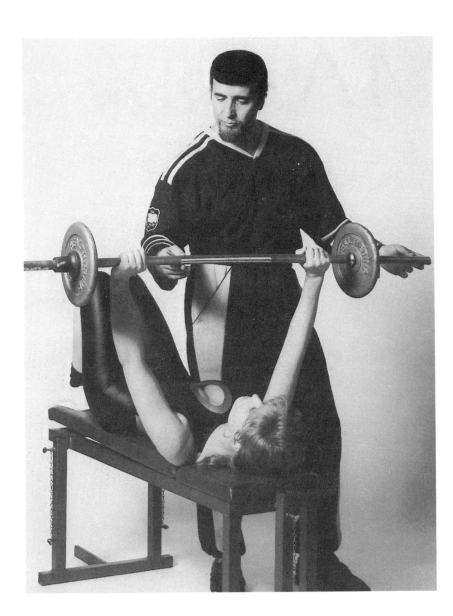

The MATRIX *Principle*

A *revolutionary approach to muscle development*

Developed in association with the Weider Research Group

Ronald S. Laura
Kenneth R. Dutton

JOHN
MAGEE
INC.

To my brother James F. Laura, whose interest in the sport of bodybuilding served to inspire my own involvement in weight training, and to whose guidance is owed whatever success I have achieved in the 'world of iron'.

Ronald S. Laura

Copyright © 1992 By John Magee, Inc.
65 Broad Street, Suite 400
Boston, MA 02109
Fax 617-695-1436
Tel 617-955-1992
    800-822-3007

Previous Editions Copyright
© R. S. Laura and K. R. Dutton, 1991

First published in 1991
Allen & Unwin Pty Ltd
8 Napier Street, North Sidney, NSW 2059 Australia

Library of Congress
Cataloguing-in-Publication entry:
Laura, R. S. (Ronald S.)
    The Matrix Principle.
    Catalog #92-60316
    ISBN: 0-910944-02-4

The Matrix Principle was developed in
association with the Weider Research Group

Set in Times New Roman 10.5 on 12 pts by Times Graphics, Singapore

The authors have great faith in this programme but cannot take responsibility for injury caused to readers. As with any exercise programme, it should be undertaken with care and with individuals working at their own pace. Seek your doctor's advice to ensure that you are in good health before embarking on this programme.

Printed in the United States of America
By Quantum Printing Corporation
Laconia, N.H.

Contents

Acknowledgments

The authors wish to express their appreciation to those who assisted with the production of this book.

Our special thanks go to Gai Gardner for her patient and careful work in typing the manuscript, to Eileen O'Donohue for her assistance with the illustrations, to Michael Lynch for equipment, and to Kim and Peter Emsermann for the photography.

We are grateful to the following, who appear in the photographic illustrations: Melissa Croft, Scott Elsley, Kim Emsermann, Peter Emsermann, Michael Gillies, Paul Haslam, Monica Haslam, Paul Henderson, Peter Hudson, Roger Ilitch, Coral Johnston, Suzanne Kondraci, Dean Kyrwood, Adam Laura, Helene Laura, Rebecca Laycock, Andrew Lewer, Jason Low, Anita Martinelli, Steven Meakes, Richard Mu, Ian Riley, Jamie Roberts, Chris Sluiter, David Soo, Lauro Sottovia, Edward H. Stephens, Marysha Stephens and Tony Webber.

Finally, we express our gratitude to Coral Johnston for the workout gear specially designed for this book. These and other items of exercise and leisure wear are available from the Corston–Mr Universe Collection, PO Box 39, Wickham, NSW, 2293 Australia, (049) 621 295, Fax (049) 622 305.

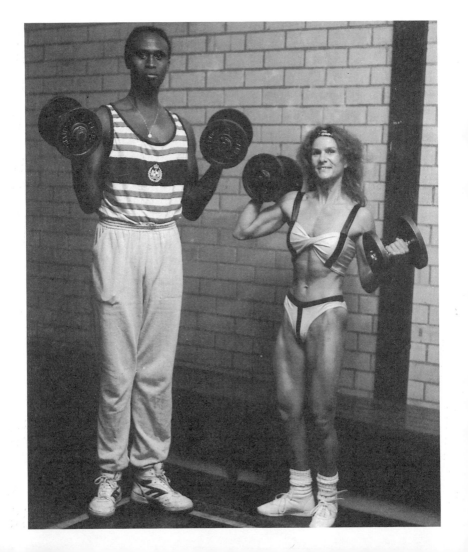

Introduction

This book introduces a radically different approach to weight training from that found in most existing works on the subject.

Until now the most comprehensive guides to the achievement of muscular development have generally been found in works aimed at either practising or potential bodybuilders. The assumption that other sportsmen and sportswomen do not benefit from bodybuilding routines, based on the old and now discredited myth of the musclebound body-builder, has usually meant that manuals of sports training, if they deal with weight routines at all, discuss them only in a cursory and prescriptive way. A number of standard weight exercises may be recommended, but only as an adjunct to training in specific sporting skills and generally without any serious discussion either of the means by which this form of training actually produces muscle growth, or of the relative effectiveness of the various training methods in fostering this growth.

In recent times, however, the importance of well-developed and efficient muscularity for sporting performance, not only in 'strength' sports such as football, discus and the like, but also in 'explosive power' sports such as sprints and short-distance swimming, has become widely recognised, and numerous sportspeople and trainers are beginning to look to muscle-building exercise as a central element of the training process. The question of the relative effectiveness of different weight-training routines in promoting muscle growth is no longer of interest to body-builders alone. This book, then, is directed both at bodybuilders and sports trainers as well as at those who wish to maximise their muscle gain whilst engaged in general fitness programs. It aims to provide a detailed treatment of the physiology and chemistry of muscle growth, in the belief that the benefits of training are most effectively gained through an *understanding* of the processes called into play when the muscles are subjected to growth-oriented exercise regimes.

But our aim goes well beyond this. Our purpose is to present an entirely new principle of weight training which has been subjected to controlled clinical tests for over a decade and has proved itself at least twice as effective in promoting muscle growth as any of the conventional training routines suggested in the standard literature on the subject. We have called this principle the *Matrix Principle*.

The Matrix Principle involves a systematic series of programs for each body-part. The word 'matrix', which we have used to describe each set of inter-related exercises, is usually defined as the particular environment within which a thing originates or develops. In simple terms, it can be defined as an array of elements which functions as a system, the interconnection of these elements being fundamental to the way in which the system works as a whole. In the sense in which it is used in this book, the term refers to the array of exercises (each devoted to a specific body-part) which are combined in particular sequences and in given modes to provide a self-contained workout for the body-part in question. Each muscle or body-part, with its surrounding array of exercises, thus becomes a matrix. This can be represented diagrammatically as follows:

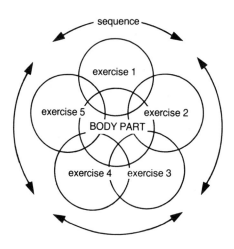

Each Matrix routine is organised in seven stages in order to accommodate the varying needs, ages and levels of fitness of weight trainers from the relative beginner to the professional bodybuilder.

Crucial to the approach adopted is a belief in the interconnection of health and fitness-related factors which affect the body's capacity for muscular growth. One way of expressing this understanding is to refer to it as a *holistic* approach to physical development. The word 'holistic' is much in vogue at present, though its meaning is not always well understood by those who use it. Briefly, we are committed to a notion of human health and well-being which seeks to restore that total view of the human organism which has become obscured by the increasing compartmentalisation of the bio-sciences (and the sciences generally) over the last three centuries or so. We believe it is time to return to an appreciation of biological phenomena, particularly at the human level, as an interconnected *system*.

In the specific terms of the present book, the concept which underpins our approach to maximum effectiveness in physical training is one which stresses the latter's role as part of a matrix of health-related factors which may again be illustrated in diagrammatic form:

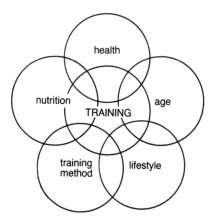

For this reason, it is strongly recommended that the reader should study the earlier chapters before passing on to the specific Matrix training routines set out in Part IV. Much of this preliminary material may already be familiar to some readers, and certain of them (e.g. those with a strong academic background in anatomy, physiology or nutrition) may find that it adds little that is new to their store of knowledge. In general, however, our experience has been that the vast majority of those undertaking weight training do so in the absence of any substantial degree of understanding of precisely *what it is that happens when they exercise*: they are given a program, which they follow on the basis of the (presumed) superior knowledge of their trainer or the author of their training manual, but they are often not aware of, and do not seek to enquire about, the causal link between the activity they engage in and the desired effect.

It is our contention, on the contrary, that an understanding of the processes involved in muscular development is not merely interesting or optional background; rather, it is crucial to advanced development. Unless the trainer can become *self-directed*—an observer of progress, a diagnostician of problems, an experimenter with new methods—then he or she will either cease to progress or will remain forever the 'pupil' of some external authority. As professional educationists, we are convinced that any educational experience should lead to the freedom which comes from knowledge, not the subservience which attaches to ignorance.

The Matrix Principle has already been subjected to exhaustive testing (see box following) and has shown itself capable of producing degrees of muscle growth of a kind previously associated only with the use of anabolic steroids. Our holistic approach to health and fitness has led to a total rejection of drugs and other artificial ergogenic aids as a means of encouraging muscular development.

Testing the Matrix Principle

The clinical tests of Matrix training were carried out in two locations: Harvard University Fitness Center, Cambridge, Mass., 1980–81 and 1984–85; and Ultra-Health and Fitness Clinic, Newcastle, Australia, 1979–80, 1982–83, 1986–90. Although assistant instructors were utilised in both locations, the research study was organised and supervised by Professor R. S. Laura. The research was clinically based in that a rigorous program of comparison between conventional and Matrix training techniques was implemented, using two to three control groups within each trial. Six trials were conducted over a period of nearly twelve years. The progress of all groups was carefully monitored; three trials were conducted for the duration of three months, three other trials were conducted over a period of six months.

Within the time frame of nearly twelve years, 162 subjects were involved in the clinical trials, though only 108 subjects actually completed the full program, comprising 84 males and 24 females. The test results reflect only the results of those who completed the program with not more than three absences out of fifteen course sessions for the three-month trial, and not more than five absences out of thirty sessions for the six-month trial. Each control group consisted of four to six subjects, usually of similar age and fitness category. Comparisons were made only between groups in which the subjects were roughly equivalent in training experience, fitness levels, age and sex.

Considerable efforts were made to ensure that all test conditions and other relevant conditions of influence were identical. Control outside the clinical sessions extended to diet, additional exercise and rest.

Three criteria of assessment were used as a basis of comparison. All subjects kept a training diary in which their variations of weight, critical measurements and strength gains were all recorded weekly. Critical measurements included: shoulder girth, chest, waist, arms, thighs and calves. Strength gains were measured for five exercises using maximum lifts for five repetitions. The five exercises were: the leg press, barbell bench press, lat machine pulldown, biceps curl, and the roll press. On average five out of six subjects in the Matrix groups showed gains in both size and strength significantly greater than in the conventional group. Some gains in size made by the Matrix groups at the completion of the course were as much as three times the gains made by the conventional group. Similarly, gains in strength by the Matrix group surpassed those of the control conventional group by a factor of 2 to 1. For every strength gain of five kilos made by the conventional groups, the Matrix groups exhibited gains of ten kilos.

We hope that, by now publishing in a single volume the material previously available only in a number of journal articles and through our personal training sessions, we shall enable many more sportspeople and bodybuilders to join the ranks of those who have found Matrix training the most effective natural means of achieving full muscular potential.

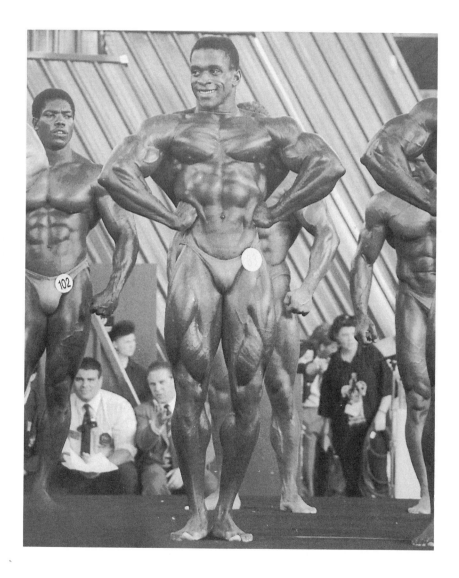

Part I

The muscle system at work

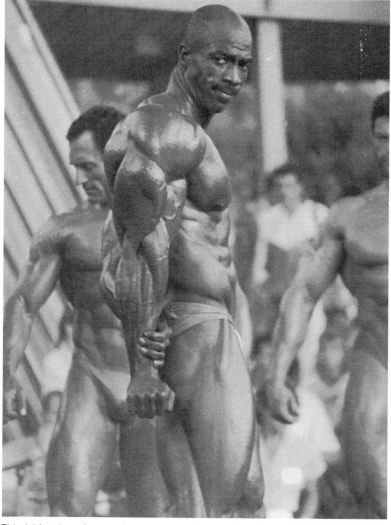

This 'side triceps' pose demonstrates the massive size attained by the triceps in a professional bodybuilder.

1   Muscle mechanics

'What exercise should I do to develop my shoulders?'

This question, and many others like it, will be familiar to every instructor. And all learners, at some stage or other, have put a similar question to their instructor or sought such information from their training manual. It is probably as good a question as any with which to introduce the subject of this chapter. How do we go about answering it?

The usual approach adopted is the most direct one. That is, a number of specific exercises will be prescribed, each of them to be performed for a certain number of repetitions and an assigned number of sets. This is, no doubt, the information the learner is seeking, and the instructor or manual provides a direct answer to the enquiry. In that sense, there is nothing wrong with the answer that is given, assuming that the instructor is reasonably well qualified and the exercises are appropriate, and the learner will undoubtedly benefit.

But if we look at the learning principle involved in this approach, we will see that it is basically unsatisfactory. For one thing, it fosters the simplistic view that muscle growth just 'happens' as a result of certain prescribed actions, and completely neglects our understanding of *why* it happens; that is, the relationship between cause and effect. For another, it works on the unjustified assumption that there is one 'correct' answer to the question asked, regardless of stage of development, age, body-type or, most importantly, the training method adopted.

Suppose, for example, that the learner has asked how many sets of a prescribed exercise should be performed, and that the instructor replies 'Three'. No doubt the answer will have been given in good faith, on the basis of the trainer's experience. But what if the questioner were to follow the instructor's answer by the further question: 'Why three? Why not two, or five, or ten?' If the 'instructor', in this case, were a standard training manual, no explanation would usually be provided and most 'live' instructors would be hard put, if pressed, to justify their original answer in any but the most general terms; that is, that this is what seems to work best.

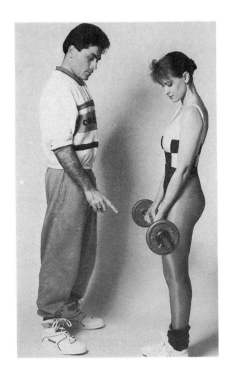

Effective weight-training instruction involves more than just teaching exercise: it should encourage an understanding of how and why it works.

What this book contends is that there is another way of answering such questions—less direct, and perhaps less *immediately* helpful to the learner (who is probably, in the nature of things, seeking a 'quick fix' to his or her problem area)—but one which in the long term is likely to be a great deal more fruitful. It entails the learner gaining an *understanding* of the processes by which muscles work and by which their growth is fostered. This is a reversal of the usual pedagogical order, whereby the learner is first taught a number of exercises and carries them out obediently (if all too often without understanding, and sometimes even incorrectly). Only later, on the assumption that progress is made and the learner enjoys the training experience, does the latter sometimes go on to develop a knowledge of the anatomical and physiological basis of muscle growth.

What we want to suggest is that the sooner learners acquire an understanding of the means by which weight training actually works, the more effective their training will be for the simple reason that they can then apply their knowledge directly to their training rather than just carry out a set of instructions in a mechanical way. In short, they will be in a position to answer their own questions. If they do seek information from an instructor or manual, they will at least know whether the answer given does or does not make sense. As we said in the Introduction, we believe this to be the proper goal of education: not to issue dogmatic instructions, but to provide the information which leads to understanding.

The Matrix Principle is based on the most recent advances in exercise physiology. It is, of couse, possible to perform the Matrix exercises outlined in Part IV without an understanding of the physiological processes on which they are based, and no doubt some trainers will be content to do so. It is our belief, however, that weight training is best undertaken on the basis of an understanding of why and how it operates to promote muscle growth, and for this reason the scientific basis on which the claim of superior effectiveness of Matrix training is made will be a recurring theme throughout the early chapters of this book.

We can now return to the question with which this chapter started, and which we can use as an illustration of how an 'educational' rather than a 'prescriptive' approach might go about answering it. The first area of enquiry that we, as instructors, would wish to explore with the learner would probably be that of the mechanical processes involved in muscle action. This takes us directly into the field of muscular anatomy and the first thing that the learner might be asked to clarify is what is meant by the 'shoulders'. If we look at Figure 3, for example, we will see that the term 'shoulders' might refer to one, or both, of two major muscles or muscle-groups, the *deltoids* and the *trapezius*. If we were to question the learner in more detail, we would want to ascertain whether it was felt that the trapezius (the 'traps') was rather too flat and under-developed in the upper section (that section which is visible from the front) or perhaps that the shoulders lacked 'breadth' because of a lack of development in the deltoids. In asking the learner to specify which of the two muscle areas he or she has in mind, we are already encouraging a 'scientific' rather than a 'layman's' approach to the study of human

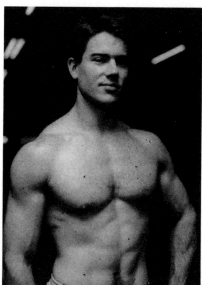

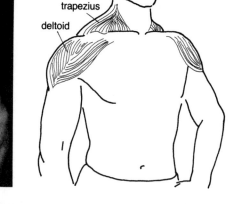

The muscles of the shoulder area

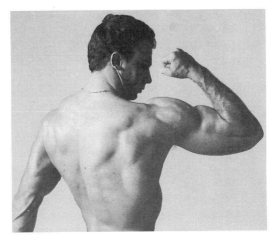

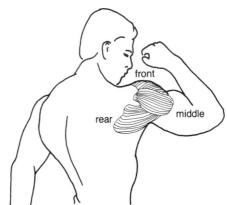

The deltoid is composed of three separate heads or bands of muscle.

anatomy and, in particular, a closer look at the location of the individual muscle-groups.

Let us suppose that the learner indicates that it is in fact the deltoids that he or she wishes to develop. What we would want to know next would be whether it is the whole of the deltoid area that is seen as needing development, or whether it is one particular 'head' of the deltoid that is the subject of concern. This, then, would lead us into a discussion of the fact that each deltoid has three 'heads', and we would need to explain that these heads are the broad bands of muscle in which the deltoids (and a number of other muscles) are arranged.

It is worth noting here that the term 'head' is the English equivalent of the Latin word *caput*, which appears in a modified form (*-ceps*) in the names of certain muscles; thus, for instance, the word *biceps* simply means 'two heads', whilst *triceps* means 'three heads'. This observation is not just an exercise in pedantry: it is a reminder that the name of a muscle, once we understand its meaning, often gives a useful and more easily memorable guide to its form or, in some cases, function. The deltoid, for example, is so named from its triangular shape which is like that of the Greek capital letter *delta* (Δ). Other muscles are named from the bone to which they are attached (e.g. the tibialis) or from the action they perform (e.g. the spinal erectors). The serious trainer is advised to learn the names of the chief skeletal muscles developed by weight exercise, as a prelude to understanding the *function* each of them performs. Brief notes on the meanings of the anatomical names are included in the Muscle Charts in the Appendix.

Our hypothetical learner, then, is invited to note that the deltoid has three separate heads, and that these are known technically as the *anterior*, *medial* and *posterior* (or, more familiarly, front, middle and rear) heads. The technical names, again, are worth noting and learning, as they often recur in describing the relative positions of other muscles or muscle-heads. We will now want to continue our questioning as to whether it is one head of the muscle or the deltoid group as a whole that the learner has in mind. For instance, the whole of the deltoid group may be perceived as underdeveloped and lacking in that roundness or fullness which characterises the advanced bodybuilder; or it may be that it is the medial head in particular that the learner wishes to develop in order to give his or her shoulders a look of greater width when seen from the front or rear.

For the sake of argument, let us suppose that it is the medial or middle head of the deltoid that the learner has in mind. Although our line of questioning has already brought us some considerable distance, from a vague reference to 'shoulders' to the identification of a particular head or band of muscle, we must now take a step back to consider a broader issue: in the present context, the issue could be posed by asking '*Why* does the deltoid have three heads?'

The question may at first seem naive, or at least unanswerable, and the instructor may be tempted to reply: 'There's no reason; it just does—that's how we are made.' While due allowance must be made for the element of truth in this answer, it can be seen on closer reflection to do scant justice to the fact that the human body is a remarkably capable machine, superbly adapted to its environment. Whether this comes about as a result of evolution or of the Creator's design is fortunately not a question that need be addressed at this stage of our enquiry: all that the learner is being asked to acknowledge is that the body is (amongst other things) a machine or mechanism each of whose parts has its specific purpose contributing to the capabilities of the whole. In the present case, we are asking our questioner to recognise that if the deltoid has three heads, then this is for a purpose (or, more accurately, three purposes).

It may seem that we are pursuing the argument to the point of stating the obvious. Unfortunately, it is a fact that the 'obvious' is all too frequently overlooked when we think about the body and its development through exercise. The point which needs to be made here, even at the risk of stating the obvious, is that the muscles have a function, and that each muscle or muscle-group *has a specific function*. Once this

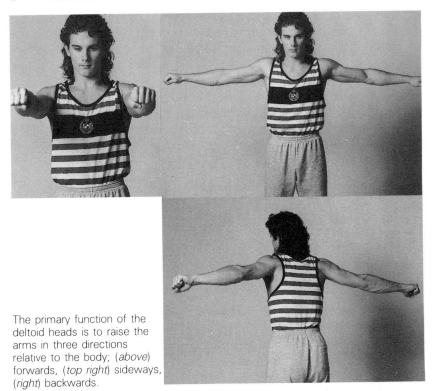

The primary function of the deltoid heads is to raise the arms in three directions relative to the body; (*above*) forwards, (*top right*) sideways, (*right*) backwards.

fundamental point has been made, we can go on to the first important principle on which a rational approach to weight training is based: namely, that *once you understand the specific function of a muscle, you can work out how best to exercise it.*

In the case of the deltoids, the function can be stated quite simply: it is to lift the arms. In more specific, but still fairly broad terms, we can say that the function of the anterior heads (or muscle bands) is to lift the arms in front of the body, that of the medial heads is to lift the arms sideways, and that of the rear heads is to pull back the arms to a position behind the body.

Such a description, of course, is very general: for one thing, it neglects the role of other muscles which may assist in these processes. But in general it is an accurate account of the chief functions of the muscles in question.

Before we explore these functions in detail, it will be helpful to consider for a moment the more general question of muscle function. In more concrete terms, it should be made clear that we are talking about one particular form of muscle, namely the 656 muscles which belong to the category known as *skeletal* muscle and make up on average 42 per cent of male and 36 per cent of female weight. There are in fact two other kinds of muscle found in the higher animals (such as humans): these are *cardiac* muscle, which is the muscle of the heart, and *smooth* muscle, which is that of the internal organs. Both skeletal and cardiac muscle are known as *striated* muscle—so named from the stripes or striations which can be seen when the muscle tissue is examined under a microscope; these striations distinguish skeletal and cardiac muscle from the so-called smooth muscle. The main difference between skeletal muscle and the other forms of muscle is that it is *under voluntary control*. For the moment, then, we can concentrate on skeletal muscle and its action, because this is the form of muscle with which weight training is concerned—the muscle that we can control at will and whose size we can increase by this form of exercise.

What we are exploring, then, is the *function* of the skeletal muscle (i.e. the mechanism by which it works and performs its specific role). As its name implies, this particular form of muscle is intimately related to the human skeleton, or the bones of the body: its function, quite simply, is to enable the body to move about, and to exert and bear forces. It does this by means of the process known as *contraction*.

The principle involved is essentially that of a system of levers and pulleys. As anyone who has studied elementary physics knows, such a system is one of the commonest in nature. Suppose that you have a fixed upright whose base is attached to a movable rod set at the horizontal, and a rope or string joining their ends: if you pull the rope so that the length joining the extremities becomes shorter, then the end of the movable rod moves closer to the end of the fixed rod.

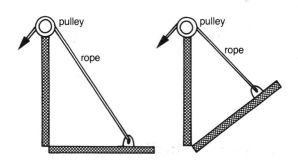

This is similar to what happens when a muscle such as the biceps contracts, except that unlike the rope, which remains of a fixed length, the length of the muscle actually decreases. In both cases, however, the two rods (in this case, the bones of the skeleton) are brought closer together.

The muscle is able to become shorter by means of its fibres bunching up; at the same time, of course, it becomes visibly thicker or more massive because of the bunching.

Skeletal muscles such as the biceps operate as what physicists call third-order levers, the fulcrum and weight being at extreme opposite ends: in the case of the biceps, the fulcrum is close to the joints, whereas the work is done at the farthest end of the lever. Since the distance between the fulcrum and the line of muscle action (known as the length

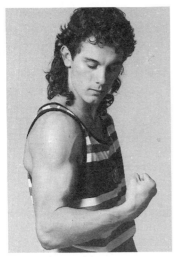
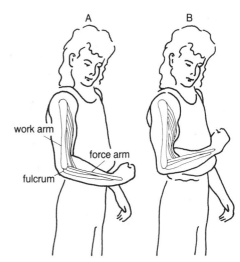

Contracting the biceps brings the lower arm closer to the upper arm.

of the *force arm*) is shorter than the length of the *work arm* (i.e. the distance between the fulcrum and the point where the work is done), this muscle works at what is called a mechanical disadvantage. This has its compensating advantages, however, as it means that a relatively short muscular contraction can produce a quick and extensive movement at the far end of the lever: thus, only a short contraction of the biceps is needed to move the forearm over a considerable distance.

We have said that the biceps operates as a third-order lever; that is to say, the muscular *effort* is applied at the insertion of the biceps into the radius bone of the lower arm and is thus between the *resistance* (the weight) and the *fulcrum* (the elbow). Other muscles operate as first-order levers (e.g. the triceps, where the fulcrum or elbow is between the resistance or weight and the muscular effort applied at the insertion of the triceps into the ulna bone); still others operate as second-order levers (e.g. the muscles of the lower leg, where the resistance or weight is between the fulcrum in the sole of the foot and the muscular effort is applied in the flexors of the foot). These types of lever are illustrated at the top of page 9.

In all of these cases, the basic principle—that of a lever as a physical device for performing work more easily—remains essentially the same: a fulcrum (the articulating surfaces of adjoining bones); a resistance or load to be moved; and a source of energy or effort (the muscles).

We have described the force exerted by the muscles as contraction (i.e. as a 'pulling' force whereby the muscles grow shorter and thicker in order to move the joints that they span). The point to note here is that the muscles have only a pulling force, not a pushing force. This force may, however, be counteracted by the load being carried by the muscle. Essentially, there are three possibilities that we can consider: a pulling force greater than the load, a load greater than the pulling force, or a

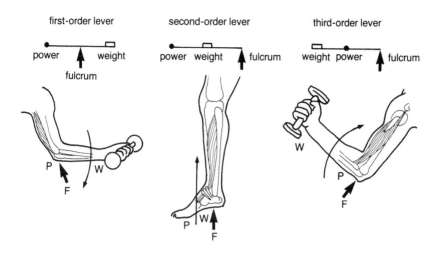

first-order lever   second-order lever   third-order lever

state of equilibrium between the pulling force and the load. These possibilities are shown in the figure below.

In diagram A, the muscle is 'stronger' than the weight or load (i.e. its pulling power is greater than the force operating against it) and the progressive contraction of the muscle will succeed in bringing the moving limb closer to the fixed limb. This is known as an *isotonic* movement, and is typical of one kind of movement used in exercise with weights: the movement from the extended to the contracted position is known as a *positive strength* or concentric contraction. In diagram B, the power of the muscle and that of the weight or load are equal, and the two limbs remain in a state of tension, with no movement: this is known as an *isometric* contraction, and it too has a function in weight-training programs. In diagram C, however, the pulling power of the muscle is not as great as the contrary force of the load; the muscle tightens, but is stretched by the external force (the weight) rather than growing shorter. Like A, this is an isotonic movement, but the movement from a contracted to an extended position is known as a *negative resistance* or eccentric contraction.

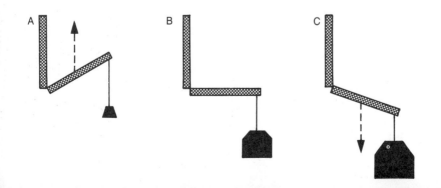

In fact, normal muscles are never completely relaxed even when they are not in active contraction: whilst they are not actively pulling, they are to some extent 'holding'—a state known as *tonus* which keeps them ready for action. For instance, the muscles of the jaw normally maintain the mandible or jaw-bone in a closed position even when we are relaxed so that the mouth does not fall open. Similarly, when we are standing up, the postural muscles (e.g. those of the leg, trunk and neck) maintain the body's posture. Only when a muscle loses tonus from injury or disease does this isometric holding of muscle tension not occur: this state is known as *muscle atrophy*. For the muscles to move the body rather than maintain it in the same position, contraction needs to occur. The effectiveness of weight training depends in the first instance on identifying the muscles that are contracted by a particular movement, and then determining what exercises can best be used to produce the desired contraction.

We can now return to the example we were discussing earlier, namely the deltoids. We can see why it is that contracting, say, the middle head of the deltoid raises the arm sideways; if no weight is held in the hands, and no other force impedes the upward movement of the arms, the force of gravity alone provides the resistance against which the muscle needs to exert its pulling power. The greater the weight or load imposed upon the arms to move them towards the ground, the greater the degree of contraction required of the deltoid to overcome this contrary force. Thus, the exercise required to 'work' the middle head of the deltoid is that which consists of raising the arms sideways against a certain degree of resistance, for example, that provided by a weight held in each hand. This is the exercise known as lateral flyes.

What if, however, the force of gravity lay in the opposite direction to that normally obtaining; if, for instance, we were hanging upside down? Since the deltoid muscles (like all others) can pull but cannot push, how could we return our arms from an outstretched position to a position close to the sides of the body since, in order for us to achieve this by the use of the deltoids, they would have to push against the force of gravity instead of pulling? To understand how this happens, we need to recognise that each muscle operates as part of a total *system*, in which other muscles come to the assistance of the particular muscle when a force opposite to the contracting (or pulling) force is required. This phenomenon is referred to by anatomists by describing the muscle in question as the *agonist* and the muscles which provide the contrary force as the *antagonist* muscles.

The simplest illustration of this combination is perhaps the biceps–triceps group. The biceps, as we have seen, is used to lift a weight by contracting and thus bringing the forearm closer to the upper arm against the weight's resistance. Suppose, however, that the weight is already lifted and needs force to lower rather than raise it. The biceps cannot perform this operation, since it cannot push the weight down but can only pull it up. The necessary function is provided by the triceps,

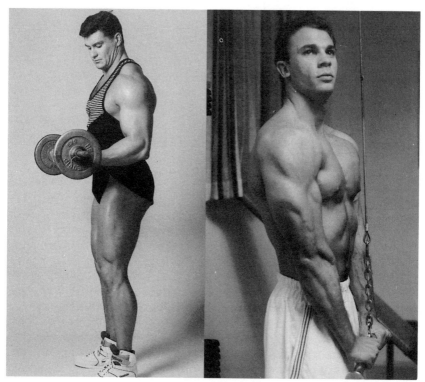

The biceps curl (*left*) flexes the upper arm, while the triceps pushdown (*right*) extends it.

which acts as the antagonist muscle to the biceps for this purpose. The biceps curl and the triceps pushdown are thus the complementary exercises.aimed at raising and lowering a weight against the resistance of the arms: the biceps is therefore sometimes referred to as a flexor muscle, and the triceps as an extensor.

The triceps contracts, thus *pulling* the lower arm into a straight line with the upper arm; in so doing, it lowers the weight by overcoming the resistance which is holding the weight up. In mechanical terms, the lever principle involved (a first-order lever) is one of extreme disadvantage, and this is one reason why the triceps needs to be a much larger muscle than the biceps. A photo of any professional bodybuilder performing the 'side triceps' pose will indicate the considerably greater size of the

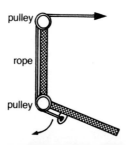

triceps than that of the biceps.

Antagonist muscles are not always found in the same body-part as the corresponding agonist muscle. In the case of the deltoid, for instance, if we were hanging upside down and wished to 'raise' our arms so that they returned to the side of the body, we should call into play a whole number of muscles of the shoulders and upper back which would act for this purpose as deltoid antagonists.

To some extent, however, antagonist muscles are involved even when the 'main' muscle is performing its normal function. Although we sometimes speak of 'isolating' a muscle by performing a movement as strictly as possible, all that we are doing is attempting to ensure that the movement involves only the target muscle and its natural antagonists, without calling on the assistance of extraneous muscles: strict biceps curls, for example, necessarily involve the triceps, whereas if not done strictly they can also call upon the assistance of the muscles of the trunk and shoulders, thus dissipating the concentration of energy.

The 'lever' model of muscle contraction is of course a simplified and schematic account of a very complex mechanical process, which involves a variety of forces operating in different combinations to produce the enormous range of movements of which the body is capable. While we have described some of the muscle operations in terms of their chief function, it is important to note that a single muscle may contract in many different patterns in order to produce a large number of different movements.

A simple experiment may help make this clear. It can be visibly demonstrated that the role of the biceps is not restricted to the lifting and 'curling' of the arm, but is also involved in the movement of the wrist. To perform this experiment, hold out your right forearm in front of you at a right angle to the body, with fist clenched and the back of the hand facing outwards, then flex the biceps as hard as possible and feel the biceps muscle with the left hand. Now turn the right fist so that the back of your hand faces downwards (as if you were curling a barbell): your left hand will feel the shape of the biceps change as its bunching pattern alters to accommodate this supplementary function. Alternatively, stand in front of a mirror and assume the bodybuilder's 'front double biceps' pose with fists clenched but the backs of your hands facing the rear. Observe the shape of the biceps. Now turn your fists so that the backs of the hands are facing outwards instead of to the rear. The changed bunching pattern of the biceps will be immediately apparent: it will appear shorter, but have a more pronounced 'peak'.

These different bunching patterns, depending on the relative angles of the body-parts to one another and the specific function being performed, indicate the complex nature of muscle mechanics, and thereby illustrate an important principle of weight training; namely, that if the muscles are to be fully exercised, they must be 'hit' or contracted *across the full range* of the positions they normally assume, in order to ensure that all muscle fibres are stimulated and that the

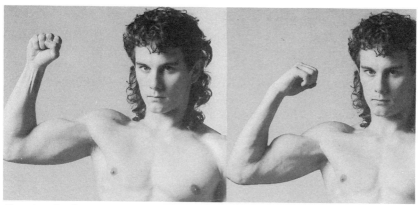

Changing the fist position alters the bunching pattern of the biceps.

whole array of antagonist and assisting muscles is called upon to the fullest extent.

This brief introduction to the mechanics of muscle contraction will have highlighted the importance of our identifying the main function performed by each muscle-group, and by specific muscles and parts of muscles within that group. Only on this basis can we concentrate our effort into a mode of performing exercises which will maximise the contraction of the particular target muscle. Though this may seem self-evident, any random sample of gym users who are asked the question 'What particular muscle is worked by the exercise you have just been doing?' will reveal an astonishingly large number of uncomprehending replies or vague approximations along the lines of: 'I was told to do it for my arms.' To exercise on the basis of anatomical ignorance will result in the trainer deriving less than optimal benefit from the effort expended, which will tend to be spread over too large a muscle area and not directed in a concentrated way on the muscle that is primarily affected.

On the other hand, we have seen that each muscle operates as part of the muscle-group or system which is called into play for any given exercise. This is known as an *interactive* system: it includes not only the primary muscle being exercised, but secondary muscles such as antagonists or assisting muscles (known as synergists). Without the multiple elements involved in this system, the movement of the limbs would be severely restricted in range and they could move through only one plane. Some of these assisting muscles (e.g. the rhomboids and infraspinatus in the upper back) cannot be worked in isolation or as primary muscles but only as part of larger groups, yet they are capable of development and need to be fully worked if the body is to achieve its full muscular potential.

What this means is that the primary muscles must be exposed to as wide a range as possible of the different movements of which they are

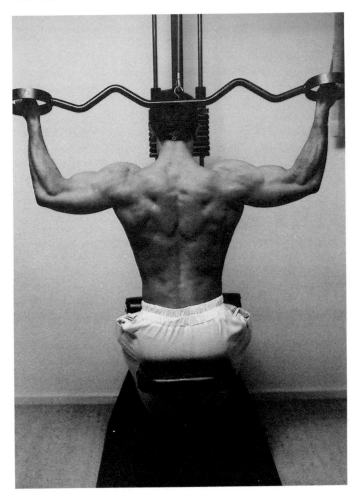

The muscles of the back form an interactive system in which some muscles cannot be worked without involving others.

capable, so as to engage the total muscle-group to the full extent. Matrix training, as we shall observe later in this book, ensures that each main muscle-group is worked through a more complete range per workout than with most conventional exercise methods, thus taking full advantage of the mechanics of muscle action. Interactive muscle-groups are stimulated to growth by interactive movements followed by isolation movements. By engaging the basic muscle-group, anabolic (or growth-directed) reactions are stimulated proportional to the area being exercised; these general anabolic reponses are then focused upon the matrix or central muscle to be exercised by the performance of isolation movements, thereby maximising the effect of the body's own anabolic functions. By this means, the benefits of interaction and isolation are combined in a unique way.

2   Muscle processes

In Chapter 1, we noted that the mechanical function of the muscles is to move the limbs by means of contraction. We now need to go on to explore the process by which this contraction takes place, since this adds an important element to our understanding of what happens when we exercise.

Before looking more closely at the skeletal muscles themselves, we should note that they are attached at one end (or sometimes both ends) to the skeleton by tendons: the outer sheath (or epimysium) of the muscle forms a common covering which provides continuity between the muscle fibres and tendon fibres. The site where a muscle is attached to an immovable (or less movable) bone is known as the *origin* of the muscle, and the site where it is attached to the more readily movable bone is known as the *insertion* of the muscle; in general, the origin is usually the end nearer the body, and the insertion the end further from the body. Between the origin and the insertion lies the *belly* or *body* of the muscle.

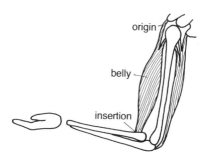

The muscle itself is composed of muscle cells or *fibres*, arranged either lengthwise or diagonally. In some cases (e.g. the biceps) the fibres run lengthwise along the muscle, while in others (such as the deltoid) they run diagonally across the muscle between two tendons which define its

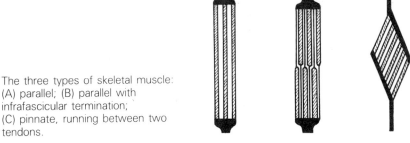

The three types of skeletal muscle:
(A) parallel; (B) parallel with
infrafascicular termination;
(C) pinnate, running between two
tendons.

edges. The biceps is therefore known as a parallel muscle whereas the deltoid, with its much shorter diagonal fibres, is known as a pinnate muscle (from the Latin *pinna*, a feather, with its diagonal pattern of barbs). This arrangement of pinnate muscles reduces the extent to which they bulge during contraction, since much of the shortening is taken up by a change in their angle of pull, which explains why the difference in size between a contracted and resting biceps is so much greater than that between a contracted and resting deltoid. In the case of parallel muscle, the fibres may run the entire length of the muscle, or only part of the way (in which case they are said to terminate infrafascicularly).

Each fibre is surrounded by a thin, transparent membrane known as the *sarcolemma* which contains both the fibrils that run the length of the fibre and link the ends of the muscles to the tendons, and also various connective tissues and membranes which respond to a variety of electrical and chemical signals. Just as each fibre is surrounded by a sheath of tissue, so the various bundles of fibres are also surrounded by a sheath (the internal perimysium) and these bundles or fasciculi are in turn grouped together and surrounded by yet another sheath (the external perimysium or epimysium). It is this latter grouping of a large number of bundles of fibres that we usually call a muscle.

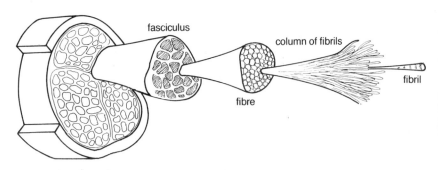

section of muscle

Muscles are made up of bundles of components, each bundle forming the element of which a larger bundle is composed.

The components of muscle fibre, and the processes they undergo, are complex, and for our practical purposes we do not need to discuss them all. Two of them, however, are worth mentioning here because of their importance in the exercise process. Firstly, the *mitochondria* are cell components in which the chemical processes necessary for muscle contraction take place. The extent to which these are present in muscle fibres varies, depending on whether the fibre tends to operate at either a steady, low level of activity or in short bursts: in the former case, the presence of a particular oxygen carrier (myoglobin) gives the muscle fibre a reddish look when seen under the microscope and it is known as 'red' as distinct from 'white' muscle fibre. The two other names used to describe this distinction are fast-twitch and slow-twitch muscle fibre, and their importance will be discussed later.

Secondly, we may note that within the muscle fibre lie groups or columns of filaments parallel to the length of the fibre. These are known as *myofilaments*, and the sets in which they are arranged are called *myofibrils*. The filaments themselves are called either thick or thin (though in fact they are all microscopically small), and their distribution is such that they overlap. During muscular contraction, this overlap of thick and thin filaments increases, as the thin filaments are drawn further and further in between the thick filaments; the effect of this is to produce the shortening or bunching of muscle fibres which is characteristic of the contracted or flexed muscle.

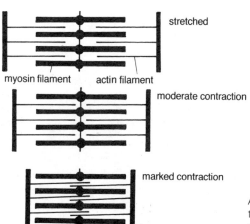

stretched

myosin filament   actin filament

moderate contraction

marked contraction

A schematic representation of the sliding filaments involved in muscle contraction.

This property of thick and thin filaments to slide over one another was not discovered until 1954; before that time it was thought that an actual shortening of the structural elements of muscle fibre took place, rather than the overlapping of filaments which do not actually change in length.

The myofilaments play an important part in the growth of muscle, known technically as *muscle hypertrophy*. Although certain factors relating to muscle growth are still not entirely clear even to scientists, the basic facts can be simply understood in terms of the body's adaptive reaction to stress.

Nature tends to respond to repeated stress by building up resistance against it, so that the next time the stress occurs it is better able to cope with it. An example can be found in the plant kingdom: controlled experiments with growing trees have revealed that if a tree is totally protected on all sides from the ambient winds, its trunk will grow to be narrower than that of a tree of the same species planted in identical conditions but exposed to the wind. Clearly, the second tree responds to the effect of winds by building a stouter trunk which will be better able to withstand the battering of occasional storms and hurricanes.

In the case of the skeletal muscles, this reaction to stress is known as the *overload principle*. A muscle subjected to repeated resistance requiring an unusual degree of effort, though not so much as to cause strain or failure, may respond by increasing in size in order to cope with this effort. For reasons still not entirely clear, this growth in size tends to occur to a greater degree when a moderate stress is repeated a number of times in succession (as happens in weight training) than when a single maximum stress is imposed on the muscles. The latter activity may increase strength but have little effect on muscle size, and this phenomenon may account for the typically more pronounced muscle size associated with bodybuilders as compared, say, to labourers engaged in hard physical work. The pumping action of the repeated contractions used in weight training causes what is known biologically as a *differentiation* (i.e. an actual change in the character of tissue), in this case in the particular form called *cellular adaptation*. This is the process by which, for example, inhabitants of high alti-

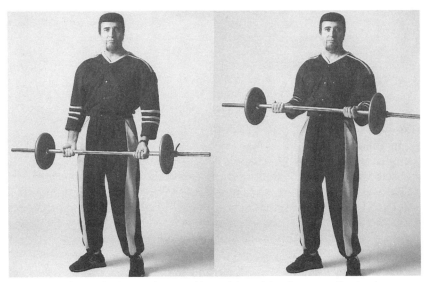

The repeated muscle contraction used in weight training is more effective in increasing muscle size than are single contractions even with heavy weights.

tudes adapt to the lowered amounts of oxygen in their environment by developing an increased number of red blood cells, thus enabling them to absorb more oxygen from the air.

What happens in muscle hypertrophy is that the myofilaments in muscle fibres, the elements which provide their contractile power, increase in number in response to the stress placed on the fibres, the purpose being to divide the work between a larger number of myofilaments. Whilst a 'normal' muscle cell might contain 2000 myofilaments, the hypertrophied cell might contain as many as 4000. The fibre as a whole thus becomes larger in diameter because of the increased number of myofilaments it contains.

For the skeletal muscles to operate in accordance with their mechanical function, the same two elements are required as is the case with man-made mechanisms; namely, a *source of energy* (to drive the mechanism) and a *signal* (to set it in motion). The energy source is of a chemical nature and is provided by substances in the body derived in large measure from the food we eat: the chemical reactions that take place in muscular contraction release energy in the forms of heat and mechanical work. We shall have more to say about this process later. For the moment, let us concentrate on the signals which bring the muscles into play.

We noted earlier that skeletal muscle is voluntary muscle (i.e. that it can be controlled at will). Just how this happens is an extremely complex process known as *neuromuscular* (or nerve-to-muscle) communication, a combination of electrical impulse and chemical reaction. Essentially, a message is sent from the brain and travels along the surface of the motor nerve cell by way of a wave of electrical changes consisting of depolarisation and subsequent repolarisation of the nerve membrane. On reaching the nerve ending, the electrical signal reaches what is knowns as a *synapse*, a junction between the nerve and the muscle in question. At this point, the nerve signal is amplified and a chemical transmitter substance known as *acetylcholine* comes into play. Its secretion is increased, and this in turn induces a change in the sarcolemma whereby receptors in the muscle fibre are electrically stimulated (or depolarised) by a redistribution of ions to produce activation of the contractile apparatus of the muscle.

In following the discussion up to the present point, you will have noticed a curious fact. In Chapter 1, we noted that the contraction of the muscle was directly related in mechanical terms to the amount of load placed upon it; what we have now discovered is that the contraction is in fact caused by an electro-chemical signal which the muscle receives *in response to* the load, *rather than by the load itself.* This fact is of considerable importance, and it means that we must now modify our earlier (purely mechanical) model of muscle contraction in favour of a rather more sophisticated model.

What happens, in effect, is that the signal received by the muscle under load is determined by the amount of the load. The amount of chemical reaction that takes place during contraction is regulated by the strength of the signal moving along the motor nerves. The obvious reason for this regulating process is to prevent the muscles from under or overreacting to the demands made upon them: if they underreact, they will not exert the force necessary to enable the limb to move when it is subjected to load; if they overreact, the limb will move too strongly and the body's energy will be used needlessly. The flow of energy, then, is subject to a complex but necessary regulatory process.

In simplified terms, what happens in contraction is that the muscle receives a series of twitches in extremely rapid succession. Each twitch is superimposed on those that have preceded it and adds to the tension, so that each twitch (known technically as a *tetanus*) is not completed before the next arrives, but is fused with the subsequent twitches to form what is known as a *complete tetanus*. If each twitch were completed before the next one arrived, we would have an incomplete tetanus, but in normal contraction the interval between stimuli is less than the contraction time: in man, a rate of 50 to 200 twitches per second (depending on the muscle involved) causes a complete tetanus or normal contraction, in which the tension steadily rises to a level plateau and remains there for a given time (until the tension is released or fatigue sets in). The maximum tension that a muscle can generate is known as its peak tetanic tension.

The strength of the stimulus will largely determine the extent of tetanus: the smallest stimulus necessary for contraction is called a *liminal* (or minimal) stimulus. This is the minimum needed for a muscle fibre to contract and it contracts completely, though the muscle as a whole does not contract, only an individual fibre does. As the load on the muscle increases, more and more fibres are called on to contract, and this accounts for the varying degrees of muscle contraction depending on the size of the load. Since not all fibres have the same 'threshold of irritability' in response to a stimulus, and not all are within the physical range of the stimulus applied, there is a wide range between the liminal stimulus and the point at which all the motor units of the muscle are brought into action (*maximal* stimulus); this intermediate range is known as *submaximal stimulus*, and is the kind of contraction which takes place when we are moving the muscles for ordinary purposes as distinct from, say, vigorous exercise with weights.

The obvious question to ask at this point is whether it is necessary to have an external force operating on the muscles in order to trigger their contraction. In other words, can the motor nerve impulses be generated without the need for a load (such as a weight) to create the stimulus against which the muscle pulls? The answer is obviously 'Yes'. Most of us will be familiar, even if we are not scientists, with the experiment whereby, say, a frog's leg muscle (e.g. the sartorius) is stimulated by a mild electric shock, and twitches or contracts in response to this stimulus. In the simplest of terms, we can say that the frog's muscle does not 'know' the origin of the electrical signal: it reacts in the same way whether the signal is generated in response to an actual load or whether it is artificially induced.

Although the effect of electrical signals upon muscle action has been known by scientists since the 18th century, it is only in recent times that this knowledge has been put to practical use; for instance, a team of scientists in Cleveland, Ohio, has recently developed a surgically implantable electrical system which enables quadriplegics, who have lost muscle function in their limbs because of spinal injury, to stimulate 'artificially' the muscles which are no longer receiving signals from the brain. Low levels of electric current are applied to the nerves by means of electrodes sewn on to the muscles in a way precise enough to activate them to produce the exact function required to perform specific tasks (e.g. grasping a pen or a can). By means of this system, known as functional electrical stimulation, quadriplegics can use various different shoulder movements to trigger specific signals in an implanted controller about the size of a pacemaker, and each type of signal produces the particular combination of muscle stimulations required to perform a particular movement.

Electrostimulation has also been used at times by bodybuilders: electrodes are applied externally to both ends of a muscle and a current is conducted through the muscle which is then led to contract and, subsequently, to knot up into a cramp. This technique, however, involves higher voltages than in the cases mentioned above since the muscles need not only to be triggered but forced to contract fully. Despite some reported successes with this method of muscle stimulation, it is not recommended because of the potential danger of a tear or strain, and in general it has not caught on as a muscle-building technique.

The point shown by these experiments is that an actual load is not necessary to bring about muscle contraction; all that is needed is a signal sent from the brain and communicated to the muscle. Skeletal muscle is, as we have observed, voluntary muscle. When we lift our forearm—for instance, to touch our shoulder with our fingers—we produce a certain amount of submaximal contraction in the biceps. We can, however, deliberately flex the biceps (without the aid of a weight) so that the degree of contraction is, if not maximal, at least much greater than that required merely to lift the arm. What we are doing, in fact, is mimicking the effect of a heavy external force against which the biceps pulls to near-maximal extent. The brain has learnt how to send to the biceps muscle the same signal that it would send if we were deliberately trying to lift a weight in the movement known as a curl. As in the case of the electrically-stimulated frog muscle, the muscle itself does not 'know' the reason for the message it receives (i.e. whether the movement is required as a response to a load, or whether the stimulation of the muscle has some other cause) yet the response is the same; namely, a significant degree of contraction.

Whether the hypertrophy (muscle growth) resulting from certain patterns of contraction derives from the tension itself, that is, from the

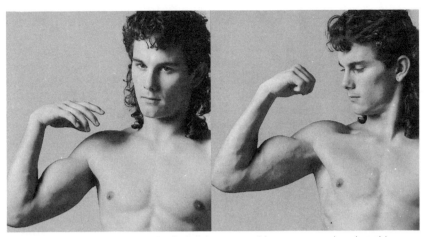

Touching the shoulder automatically involves some biceps contraction, but this can be increased at will to produce the maximal contraction known as flexing.

physical properties of the muscle fibres (myogenic factors), or whether it is a result of the motor neurone impulses which cause the contraction to occur (neurogenic factors), has been the subject of some debate amongst physiologists. The present state of research suggests that a combination of neural and biomechanical factors may be the controlling mechanism. It is probable that the rate of protein synthesis is affected by the concentration of sodium and (especially) calcium ions, and that the source of this metabolically important signal is slight surface depolarisation of the muscle membranes. Since this depolarisation can be induced by either a barrage of nerve impulses or a change in membrane permeability caused by stretch, it seems probable that both nerve-evoked and stretch-induced factors play a part in the metabolic stimulation leading to hypertrophy.

We noted earlier that contraction involves two types of muscle fibre, usually known as white or fast-twitch fibres and red or slow-twitch fibres. Fast-twitch fibres characteristically generate maximum tension in about one-third the time required by slow-twitch fibres, and produce about twice the amount of contractile force. However, although these white or fast-twitch fibres exhibit rapid and strong contractile responses, they display correspondingly rapid fatigue patterns. The reason for this is that the energy flow of a muscle fibre is roughly proportional to its energy dissipation; thus, as the speed of muscle contraction increases, the force of muscle contraction decreases. The red slow-twitch fibres, on the other hand, have a much greater capacity for *sustained* effort: the myoglobin which gives the slow-twitch fibres their reddish hue considerably enhances the fibre's endurance capacity and ability to perform sustained work with submaximal loads.

What does this mean in practice? In fact, it means a great deal in terms of the effect produced by different training methods. The aim of weight training for muscle development is to produce muscle hypertro-

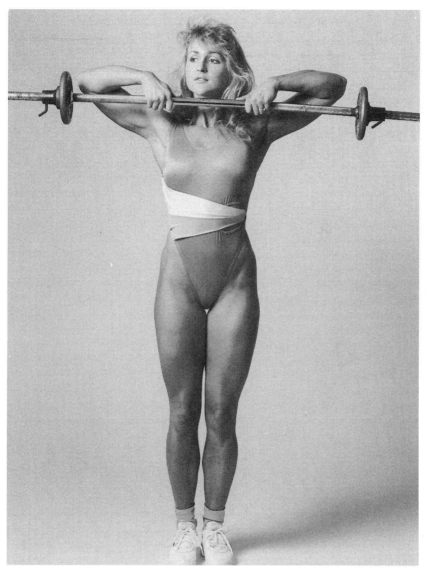

Heavy weights and low repetitions are not the only means of building muscle: light weights can also be effective if properly used.

phy (i.e. an increase in muscle size), and it will therefore concentrate on the factors likely to create this effect. Fast-twitch fibres show a greater capacity for hypertrophy than slow-twitch fibres, since the size and number of fibres contained in fast-twitch units are greater than in slow-twitch units: this factor, which accounts for the more significant output of force characteristic of fast-twitch fibres, leads exercise physiologists to link muscle growth directly with fast-twitch fibre stimulation. Since *low repetitions* are presumed to promote the development of the myofibrillar elements associated primarily with the growth pattern of fast-twitch fibres, and *high repetitions* are thought to enhance the development of cell mitochondria associated with slow-twitch fibres, the conventional wisdom makes a clear distinction between the effects of low and high repetition training.

Put simply, the conventional view is:

HEAVY WEIGHTS, LOW REPETITIONS
(fast-twitch fibre: strong, but tires) → GAINS IN MUSCLE MASS AND STRENGTH

LIGHT WEIGHTS, HIGH REPETITIONS
(slow-twitch fibre: less strong, but endures better) → GAINS IN ENDURANCE
                                                        AND
                                                        DEFINITION

There is certainly an element of truth in this view, but its equation of exercise type with the type of gains produced is far too simplistic. It is true that the use of heavy weights can promote the building of muscle mass, just as it is true that light weights can be used to improve stamina and definition. But recent physiological research has demonstrated the conventional opposition between low and high repetition training to be unnecessarily limiting. More will be said about this later, but for the moment it is important to note the growing body of evidence to suggest that it is by no means necessary to use heavy weights to increase muscle mass. It is possible, for instance, to enhance voluntarily the brain signals to the muscles which lead to contractile response, or to use exercise methods and sequences which favour the stimulation of the full range of muscle fibres.

The Matrix Principle is based on our finding that specific sequences of fast and slow repetitive movements can be used to achieve full-range fibre stimulation. In this respect, it supersedes the conventional opposition between exercise with light and heavy weights, and represents a considerable advance in training methodology.

3   Muscle chemistry

We have seen that the mechanism controlling the muscles, like other mechanical systems, functions on the basis of a set of operating instructions (or signals) and a source of energy. Having briefly discussed the signalling process in Chapter 2, we can now move on to consider the energy source. This requires at least a cursory treatment of the chemical constitution of skeletal muscle and the processes of conversion by which its activity is generated. Whilst a full discussion of these issues would involve a level of technical complexity lying outside the scope of the present work, the serious weight trainer should know enough, at least in general terms, about the metabolic factors related to muscle function in order to be able to increase to the maximum the degree of muscle growth of which he or she is capable.

Only 25 per cent of sketetal muscle consists of solid material, the remaining 75 per cent being made up of water. As to the solid material, 20 out of the 25 per cent is protein, the remaining 5 per cent being composed of carbohydrate, various organic extractives and some inorganic material. It is, then, with *protein* that we can most usefully begin this general outline.

Three proteins—*myosin*, *actin* and *tropomyosin*—make up the major part of the protein content of muscles. To return to the thick and thin muscle filaments mentioned in Chapter 2, we should note at this point that the thick filaments are composed of myosin while the thin filaments are made up of actin; myosin accounts for about half the dry weight of the contractile part of muscle, and is thus the most abundant protein present. To understand its role, it is necessary to know something about the compound *adenosine triphosphate* or ATP, which is one of the most important of the so-called 'muscle extractives' and, in particular, to know that it can be chemically converted in a process through which a large amount of energy is released. This process is achieved by the rupture of the terminal phosphate of ATP, entailing the liberation of inorganic phosphate (P) and the consequent formation of *adenosine diphosphate* (ADP).

A particular property of the protein myosin is that its molecules, by possessing the ability to create this reaction (i.e. to split ATP into ADP plus inorganic phosphate), are able to release a considerable amount of chemical energy which is converted into mechanical energy by force generators (probably the cross-bridges between muscle filaments, though this has not been clearly established). The protein actin enhances this ATP-splitting activity of myosin, and the participation of water is also required. The process is known as an energy-yielding reaction. To restore equilibrium, it needs to be followed by another reaction, which has the effect of rebuilding the ATP that is used during contraction.

Energy rebuilding takes place in two ways. One involves the muscle calling upon reserves of *phosphocreatine* (PCr) which, with the assistance of the enzyme *creatine phosphotransferase* (CPT), permits regeneration of ATP. In this reversal process, however, the muscle's supply of PCr tends to be gradually used up and therefore needs to be replenished. The recovery process is one in which foodstuffs are broken down, and this synthesis of high-energy phosphate from foodstuffs is the second element by which the energy supply is restored.

The two forms in which foodstuffs are used in the energy supply are found either as *glycogen* (a polymer of glucose) or as *fatty acids*. In the first case, known as glycolysis, oxygen is not present and glycogen is broken down in a process (the glycolytic pathway) which leads to the formation of lactic acid (glycogen $\rightarrow$ lactic acid + energy). In the second; usually known as the Krebs cycle, oxygen is present and this process is often referred to as the fatty acid oxidation cycle.

If built up in sufficient quantity, the lactic acid causes a burning sensation in the muscle area(s) being exercised. Lactic acid accumulation is also partly responsible for the sensation of 'muscle pump' characteristic of bodybuilding and other forms of intensive exercise. With the accumulation of waste substances in the muscle, the mitochondria enlarge, triggering the creation of additional capillaries or reactivating existing channels between the venous and arterial systems which expedite the dissipation of lactic acid while augmenting the supply of oxygen and nutrients to the cells. The relevant vessels dilate to accommodate the increased blood flow and the engorged muscle thus becomes enlarged.

The main problem created for the weight trainer by lactic acid accumulation is the sensation of fatigue. In fact, approximately 50 per cent of fatigue toxins are eliminated from the muscle area after a rest period of only 10 seconds, and 75 per cent flush away after 15 seconds, so that a pause in the training routine can be of great assistance. The conventional method of doing a number of sets of the same exercise, particularly if the rest period between them is minimal, can result, however, in a lactic acid build-up which is so painful that the major muscles engaged in the exercise feel totally exhausted. In consequence, subsequent movements which depend on these muscles

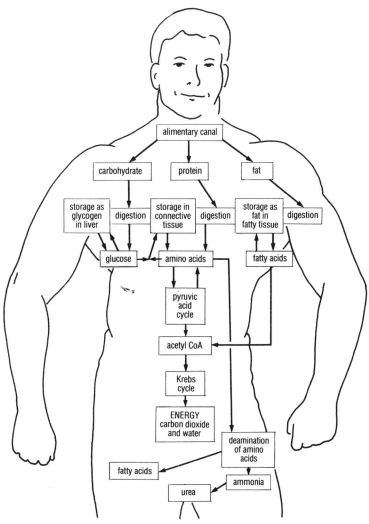

Energy intake in the form of food is converted by the body into other energy forms required for the body's maintenance and mechanical energy output.

but engage other areas of the same muscle-group cannot be activated with maximum intensity.

The Matrix Principle overcomes this problem by varying the movements within sets and the sequences of sets in such a way that the lactic acid build-up has time to dissipate to a substantial degree during the exercise of the muscle area in question, being sufficient to cause a pump but not to the point where muscle fatigue impairs the intensity of movements and reduces their effectiveness.

We can summarise the foregoing by saying that the energy released in the various chemical reactions involved in muscle contraction goes

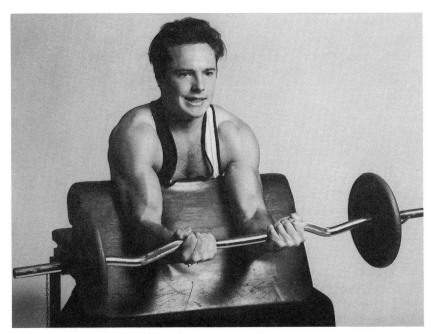

The lactic acid build-up created by repeated contraction can produce a sensation of pain and lead eventually to exhaustion.

either into the actual bunching of the muscle, or into the resynthesis of the chemical substances that participate. The excess energy liberated in all the reactions is used for heating the body, growth, and other metabolic processes taking place within the body, while the oxygen debt is repaid by respiration and other regenerative processes.

The purpose of the above brief discussion has been to provide a general guide to the chief chemical processes involved in the generation of energy by means of the muscle system. Before we can go on to consider the practical consequences of this information to the weight trainer, it will be useful to mention briefly the main types of substance which play a role in the processes described. These can be listed as:

Carbohydrates (sometimes called 'sugars' or 'starches') They provide the body with its most available source of energy, are stored in certain cells and constitute a reserve fuel supply. Carbohydrates, which are made up of carbon, hydrogen and oxygen, are divided into three groups: monosaccharides (e.g. glucose), disaccharides (e.g. sucrose) and polysaccharides (e.g. glycogen, which is found in muscle).

Lipids and fats Again, these contain only carbon, hydrogen and oxygen, but because they contain more carbon and hydrogen than do carbohydrates they can combine with many more units of oxygen to provide much more heat energy per unit weight. Fats are compounds of saturated or unsaturated fatty acids, and lipids are generally esters of fatty acids. Related to the fats are sterols or sterids (e.g. cholesterol, ergesterol, sex hormones and D vitamins). Hydrocarbons (which include certain vitamins) are classed as lipids, as are neutral fats which are esters of fatty acids with glycerol. Fats are well known for their high caloric value.

Proteins   These also possess carbon, hydrogen and oxygen, but additionally they contain nitrogen and usually sulphur. Proteins are made up of amino acids (fatty acids in which a hydrogen atom has been replaced by an amine group). Proteins are the main material of animal tissue, and act as growth material. In the growth of muscle tissue, for instance, additional proteins are formed from the amino acids taken from the blood. The end products of protein metabolism include creatine, which is required (in the form of phosphocreatine) for muscle contraction.

Enzymes   These act as catalysts (i.e. they increase the speed of a reaction without being used in the reaction itself) and assist in the chemical changes that occur in the metabolic activity of the cells. We have seen that the enzyme CPT is involved in the regeneration of ATP.

Nucleic acids   These are necessary for protein synthesis in the body. The best known is deoxyribonucleic acid or DNA, the means of storing genetic information in living cells.

Other substances   These of course include water (which acts both as a solvent and as a medium of transfer), as well as various mineral substances (e.g. calcium ion, potassium, magnesium, sodium ion, phosphate, carbonate and sulphur). In general, their role is to maintain the acid–base equilibrium and to help in the release of energy. They are also important in forming compounds (such as hormones) which help regulate cellular activity.

The aim of the above summary guide, and the preceding general description of chemical activity in the muscles, is not to provide a complete account of the complex chemical make-up and processes of the body. Its purpose is rather to indicate to the weight trainer something of the multitude of factors which are called into play both in the body's routine functioning and, more particularly, in the exercise of the muscle system. In the context of the present work and its approach, what it demonstrates is that the chemical processes of muscle contraction involve numerous interactions of chemical components, only some of which take place within the muscles themselves while others are produced within different internal organs. The importance of maintaining a balanced food intake, and the various means of enhancing the chemical processes involved in muscle growth, will be discussed in more detail in Part II.

A holistic approach to weight training will emphasise that the effects of exercise are best realised when they are part of a total regime of energy throughput which also includes appropriate food intake, and that these effects can be further increased by appropriate and natural forms of diet supplementation. Part III of this book examines how diet can be

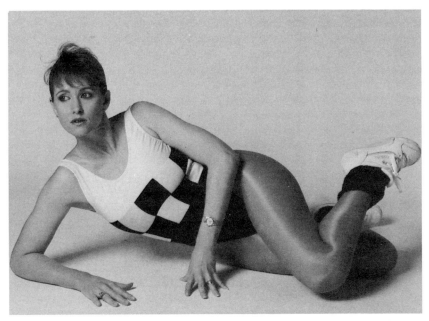

Like weight training, aerobic exercise requires adequate nutrition of the muscle system.

controlled to work in conjunction with Matrix training in order to reduce obesity whilst maximising the growth of lean muscle.

4   Muscle size

Many people who embark on a program of weight training suffer from a popular misconception. Unfortunately, it was given widespread currency some years ago by the advertisements placed in magazines by one of the most successful promoters of muscle development of all time: Angelo Siciliano, who called himself 'Charles Atlas'. The Charles Atlas advertisement which gained most celebrity was that of the 'seven-stone weakling' who found when he appeared on the beach that bullies kicked sand in his face. After a course of Charles Atlas' 'Dynamic Tension' method of muscular development, the puny victim found himself transformed into an impressively developed bodybuilder who excited the envy of other men and the admiration of attractive women. The advertising campaign, which ran for many years and was widely emulated by other promoters of bodybuilding equipment and exercise methods, played successfully on the aspirations and feelings of inferiority experienced by many who saw, or could be persuaded to see, their lack of physical development as a sign of personal inadequacy. Although it made Charles Atlas a very wealthy man, the campaign regrettably left behind it a large number of unhappy people who found that the remarkable results promised failed to eventuate in their particular case. Nonetheless, the myth persists in a number of forms even today, including what might be called its 'reverse' form.

Many of those who present themselves for a course in weight training are anxious to establish early in their exercise program that they do not want to become 'too muscly': 'I don't want to end up looking like Arnold Schwarzenegger' is a comment frequently heard by weight-training instructors the world over. It is hard to know where to begin in order to assure these beginners that they certainly run no risk of such outstanding results from the modest course in which they intend to engage. It is probably fruitless to explore with them the psycho-sexual complex which makes the sight of a world-class professional bodybuilder appear to some people not only unattractive but positively repugnant, although this is in itself a fascinating field of psychology. It is probably much better to tell them the simple but inescapable truth: to attain, and then maintain, such a degree of muscularity, definition, symmetry and proportion they would need to engage in years of gruelling training, involving hours per day most days of the week; to push themselves beyond excruciating pain barriers, maintain demanding schedules of weight gain and weight loss, master the intricacies of posing and presentation and, *even then*, they might never get beyond the point reached by the thousands of would-be competitive bodybuilders who never reach a placing in competition.

The fact is that the development of muscle size is not achieved easily. All human beings are of course endowed with muscularity. We all have the same number of muscles, and all reasonably healthy humans possess a muscular system which works with remarkable efficiency. In most cases, it is more than adequate for the manifold physical tasks involved in everyday living: walking, running, lifting, pushing, pulling, jumping, stretching and so on. While some people perform these functions more easily than others, depending on their degree of general fitness, the presence or absence of obesity and of various physical impairments (e.g. from injury or disease), it is obvious that the 'average' person manages to cope quite adequately on the basis of a muscular system which is kept in working order by the normal functions of mobility without being developed to an outstanding degree.

While this observation holds true in a general sense, it is equally notable that a cross-section of almost any group of adult humans will usually reveal considerable individual differences—not only of height, weight, body fat and facial characteristics, but also of muscular development. And in many cases this latter characteristic will relate as little to behavioural factors (e.g. the amount of exercise actually performed in daily life) as do their other physical characteristics. In other words, some people (including certain racial groups) just seem to possess a degree of 'natural' or 'innate' muscularity which others do not.

This phenomenon is sometimes experienced by weight trainers as dispiriting and discouraging. Try as they may, and despite frequent hard workouts, they just cannot escape the fact that they are 'naturally thin', or that if they eat as their appetite dictates their food intake turns to fat rather than muscle. They often wonder what they are doing wrong, and may be tempted to give their exercise program away completely.

Unfortunately, there is no simple remedy that can be proposed to those who are in this situation. And certainly the miraculous transformations we talked of earlier—those sometimes promoted by the purveyors of bodybuilding courses or exercise equipment—will prove little more than an elusive fantasy. More realistic levels of muscle growth are certainly possible, and indeed achievable given perseverance and appropriate types of exercise, but the fact remains that we are to a large extent (though fortunately not entirely) the prisoners of our natural *somatotypes.*

For those readers who are not familiar with somatotyping, a few words will be appropriate here. It is a method of classifying physical shape, based on the work in 1940 of the American psychologist William H. Sheldon. It does not measure size, though interesting results can emerge from the correlation of certain body-types with size. As a psychologist, Sheldon was primarily interested in the relationship between body-structure and personality, though his work is also of interest in the study of psychomotor skills, voice-type variations and a variety of physiological data. He postulated three extremes of body shape, namely:

- The *endomorph*: a rounded body with round head, bulbous stomach, heavy build and relatively high proportion of body fat;
- The *mesomorph*: broad shoulders and relatively narrow hips, and a high degree of bone and muscle relative to fat;
- The *ectomorph*: narrow shoulders and hips, thin arms and legs, little muscle or fat, and a large skin area relative to total bulk.

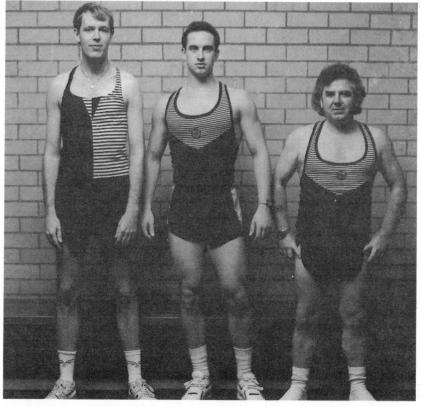

Some body-types display a relatively marked degree of ectomorph, mesomorph or endomorph characteristics.

Two points should immediately be made in relation to this classification. Firstly, the basic body shape is 'given' and does not change significantly with diet: a starved endomorph does not become an ectomorph but retains the same basic body shape; an overfed mesomorph may look (and in fact be) fat, but will still tend to look powerfully-built; and an ectomorph may develop a 'gut' but still retain a basically spindly look in the limbs. Secondly, the classification recognises that the components listed tend not to occur in a 'pure' form but in varying degrees in different people. Thus, a person with extremely pronounced endomorphy might conceivably score 7 (the highest rank) on Sheldon's endomorph scale, and 1 (the lowest rank) on the mesomorph and ectomorph scales. This type of physique, which occurs rarely if at all, would be written as 711. Similarly, an extreme mesomorph would be classed as 171 and an extreme ectomorph as 117. The person of presumed 'medium' physique is classed as 444. Most of us, however, will have different scores on each scale, so that we will be ranked as 521, 226, and so on. The classification numbers (or scores) are negatively correlated, so that a high number in one class precludes high numbers in the others.

It should be noted that no one body-type is associated with high athletic ability: ectomorphs who are tall and lean often make good oarsmen, fencers or basketball players, for instance, while champion wrestlers (especially Sumo wrestlers!), shot putters and some weightlifters are usually thick-trunked and short-limbed endomorphs. The broad-shouldered and slim-hipped mesomorph type is often found amongst swimmers, gymnasts and pole-vaulters and of course many, though by no means all, top bodybuilders also fit into this classification.

Despite its relative subjectiveness and a certain lack of subtlety, Sheldon's somatotype system is still widely used and is a helpful means of looking at the variety of physique types. Other factors must of course be considered if a total picture of human body-types is to be formed: height, for instance, is a major determining factor, and while this may tend to cluster around certain extremes in particular groups (e.g. the African Watusi with an average male height of 196 cm (6ft 5in), or the African pygmies at the other extreme), its distribution is generally more varied throughout the world.

Much work is still being done in the correlation of physical type with athletic performance in certain sports. The typical Olympic weightlifter's physique (even in the lightest weight division) is so different from that of the average marathon runner that the correlation of physical type with outstanding performance in certain sports is obvious to all.

As far as strength sports are concerned, there are obvious reasons why pronounced ectomorphs may be less proficient performers than mesomorphs or endomorphs. This is a simple matter of muscle mechanics, and of differences in the ratio between the force and work arms of the levers involved: we need only consider the difference between a race-horse (with its long legs, or work arms) and a burrowing animal such as a mole (with its very short limbs and muscles) to understand the difference between a mechanical system aimed at maximum speed and one aimed at maximum strength. For this reason, the length and thickness of the bones, particularly in the limbs, is often a guide to the amount of muscular force favoured by the physique, the circumference of the wrist being sometimes used as a rough guide.

It is not simply the length and thickness of bones which vitally affect the capacity for muscular effort. The physical disposition of muscles, in terms of the distance of their insertion from the joints about which the bones (or levers) move, can be a critical factor in increasing mechanical advantage and thus performance. Two men of similar weight, build and age will display an enormous difference in the effort they require to curl a 16 kg (35 lb) dumbbell where one has a 'long' insertion of the biceps on to the radial tuberosity of the lower arm (7.5 cm or 3 inches from the fulcrum or elbow-joint) and the other a 'short' insertion (2.5 cm or 1 inch from the elbow). On the assumption that they both have 40 cm (16 inch) long resistance arms, the 'effort' required by the first man is 85 kg (187 lb) while that required by the second is 256.6 kg (564.5 lb). The mechanical advantage provided by a difference of five centimetres (two inches) in the distance at which the biceps is inserted on the radius enhances the effective strength of the muscle to such a degree that the effort the first man requires to curl a 16 kg (35 lb) dumbbell is 171.5 kg (377.5 lb) less than that of the second man. It is obvious, then, that the bone–muscle configuration will play a critical role in the capacity for weight training, and that it must be added to the list of genetically determinant factors.

Other relationships, however, remain more elusive; for instance, why the success of black athletes in sports such as track and field athletics has not hitherto been matched by their success in presumably similar kinds of sport such as swimming. Questions of training opportunity may of course be involved, but only continuing research by exercise physiologists will be able to provide definitive answers.

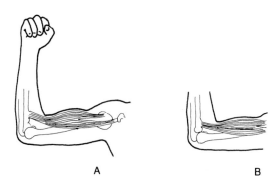

A   B

The insertion of the biceps muscle into the radius bone: (A) long insertion; (B) short insertion

Somatotyping, then, does much to enable us to understand the likely physical abilities of various body-types (e.g. the improbability of a 711 endomorph becoming a successful long-distance runner), but essentially it is a means of classification rather than an explanation of physical type. For the explanation, we would need to look to the field of genetics, and in particular to the role of nucleic acids as transmitters of genetic information in the cell and as a necessary element in protein synthesis in the body.

Nucleic acids are complex in structure, consisting of long chains of what are called nucleotides; one of them in particular—deoxyribonucleic acid or DNA—was not decoded until 1953 when Watson and Crick first analysed the characteristic 'double helix' structure (two interwoven helical chains of polynucleotides). The role of DNA is the encoding of genetic information and thus the transference of genetic characteristics; understanding its function is fundamental to an understanding of how our individual physical (as well as mental and emotional) peculiarities come to be as they are. Our genetic inheritance determines, amongst other things, the basic parameters of our physical capabilities, including our natural muscular configuration. The natural mesomorphs, those who approach 171 on the Sheldon scale, may do very little or no exercise: the 'code' written into their genes is such that their food intake is processed into muscle protein with little or no additional stimulus being required. The natural ectomorphs, on the other hand, send very different messages to their bodies' metabolic organs.

Racial characteristics are a further complicating factor, for they suggest genetic messages which convey a different distribution of muscularity from one racial group to another; for example, people belonging to some Asian groups (particularly Chinese) often have remarkably large and full gastrocnemius or calf muscles, whereas Australian Aborigines tend to have very little calf development so that their lower legs can look extremely thin. There are, no doubt, good reasons for these differences which may be accounted for historically but not entirely by variations in diet and patterns of work and other physical activity. The full explanation may well lie in gene codes whose messages are still showing up in the genes of distant descendants. For the moment, however, racial differences form but one more element in a genetic puzzle which hides the answer to why some people (of *all* racial groups) possess a greater potential for muscular development in some body-parts than in others. To attribute these differences to 'inherited factors' does little more than to re-position the issue many generations earlier; it does not explain the phenomenon.

The question, therefore, is whether exercise aimed at muscle development can be effective in cases other than those where the individual possesses a high degree of natural mesomorphy: the answer is 'yes'. Sheldon himself recognised that the rankings in his various somatotype categories should range, not from 0 to 7, but from 1 to 7—in other words, that there is a little of the mesomorph (and the ectomorph and

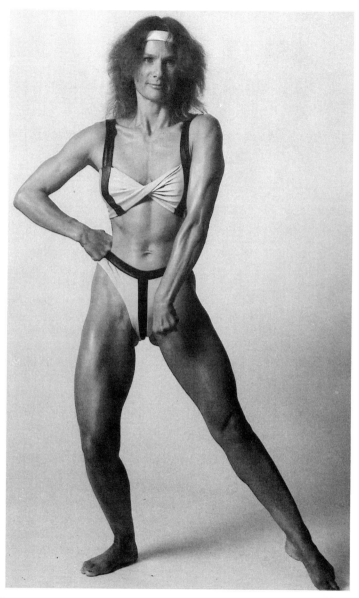

Not all successful bodybuilders (male or female) are pronounced mesomorphs: Marysha Stephens' physique exhibits a number of ectomorph characteristics, yet she has won numerous bodybuilding competitions.

endomorph) in us all. This was an observational rather than a biological finding but, to the extent that all of us have a muscle system which operates to hold our skeleton upright and allow it to move around, it is obvious that even the least 'muscular' of people have an operational muscle system, and thus possess the raw material of development. The real question, then, is whether the genetically determined messages received by our muscles can be effectively supplemented by other, learnt, messages in such a way that the muscles achieve a higher degree of growth than would otherwise be the case. Clearly, such a learning task would be greater in some cases than others—where the genetic message is weaker—and the final result would be limited by that fact. No 216 ectomorph will ever make Mr or Ms Olympia, and aspiring weight traniners must come to terms with this fact. On the other hand, not all top professional bodybuilders are extreme mesomorphs; though meso-morphy predominates in their physique, it is often accompanied by the presence of endomorph or ectomorph characteristics which would score greater than 1 on the Sheldon scale.

One point which should therefore be stressed is that trainers' goals need to be realistically adjusted in line with their natural bodily configuration as well as, of course, with their age, general physical condition and other factors. This having been recognised, learners can concentrate on achieving the *best result consistent with their body type*—the preponderantly ectomorphic can aim at developing a well-defined, lithe physique, the mainly endomorphic can combine diet and exercise so as to look powerful and robust rather than flabby, whilst the natural mesomorph can set his or her sights on a possible bodybuilding career. Once again, however, it should be noted that since very few of us score as low as 1 on the mesomorphy scale, the goal of weight training would still be to maximise our natural genetic endowment and exploit its latent potential.

We have described some of the basic parameters of muscle size and development which are 'built in' at birth, and have noted that although they may place a greater or lesser degree of limitation on the body's response to exercise, it is possible to modify them to at least *some* extent by non-artificial means in order to foster those characteristics which are more predominant in the natural mesomorph. There is, however, an additional limiting factor in muscle development which has usually been considered incapable of modification but which is currently being re-evaluated in the light of recent research. This factor is the number of muscle cells with which we are endowed at birth.

It has long been known that each of us is born with a different number of muscle cells, and that some individuals have literally millions more such cells in their bodies than do others. Since the effect of weight-based exercise is to increase the size of the muscle cells—the effect known as *hypertrophy*—it is obvious that the more cells we have available to enlarge in this way the greater will be our potential for muscular development. The orthodox view held by physiologists has been that the number of such cells that we possess is given at birth and does not change during our lifetime. Thus, bodybuilding exercise is seen as an attempt to add more size to each cell but it cannot, according to this view, change the number of cells, since this has been genetically deter--mined. Those individuals who are born with the largest number (some-times described as a full complement) of muscle cells will respond best to weight training since they have more genetic raw material to work with than those individuals with fewer muscle cells. The more muscle cells contained in the biceps, for example, the greater its potential for growth through the enlargement of the available cellular components.

There is, however, an interesting body of research which suggests that this conventional theory may need modification, and that certain forms of intensive exercise may in fact be capable of inducing an increase in the number of cells in the exercising muscle—a compensatory response known as *hyperplasia*. This effect arises, it is suggested, from the splitting of cells as a response to the need for the muscle, under certain kinds of exercise, to increase its absolute tension while maintaining an optimal speed of contraction (see William J. Gonyea, 'Role of exercise in inducing increases in skeletal muscle fiber number', in *Journal of Applied Physiology* (Respirat. Environ. Exercise Physiol.) 48, 3 (1980): 421–426).

Although the hyperplasia theory has a number of respectable advocates in the scientific community, its critics (e.g. Taylor and Wilkinson, in *Sports Medicine* 3 (1986): 190–200) point to the fact that the evidence for this process is largely indirect and that its observation in humans is open to caution on methodological grounds. Further experimentation will be needed if it is to be considered a fully substantiated theory. Our purpose at this point is chiefly to indicate the far-reaching consequences which would follow from the possibility of cell splitting, in terms of the ability to overcome one of the most significant limitations imposed by our natural genetic inheritance. If the number of muscle cells could first be increased (hyperplasia) and the resulting larger number of cells then be developed to maximum size (hypertrophy), the results obtained must be considerably greater than could be achieved by hypertrophy alone.

One of the most significant advances represented by the Matrix Principle is that it uses the methods first developed by scientists working on the induction of hyperplasia in laboratory animals, and takes advantage of the results of electron microscope analysis of hyperplasia effects in control groups of athletes. These experiments have led to a number of conclusions as to the type of exercise which is most conducive to muscle growth, and these conclusions have been incorporated and exhaustively tested in Matrix weight-training programs over a decade. Not just any program of resistance training can produce this effect; the particular feature of the Matrix Principle is the combination of increased muscle tension with an accelerated rate of tension generation which has been found to be the most effective means of inducing the enhanced muscle growth noted by physiologists working on the hyperplasia theory.

5 The working system

The preceding chapters have provided a brief introduction to the complex network of inter-related factors involved in the operation of the muscles. It is important to recognise that the muscles function as one element of activity of a total *system* consisting of mechanical, chemical and neurological agents. We described this system in the Introduction in terms of a matrix, which was represented as follows:

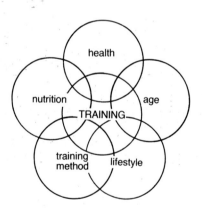

This is known as a *holistic* (as opposed to an isolationist or reductionist) view of the body's mode of functioning.

To understand fully the operation of the muscles, therefore, it is necessary to appreciate the input of the total range of stimuli which affects the muscles' ability to perform the tasks required of them. A simple example may make this clearer: a well-known experiment requires a human subject to tap a finger tip repeatedly and rapidly on a table. This activity can be kept up for a short period, but it is not long before the finger tip tires, suffers a kind of paralysis, and refuses to tap any more. If the relevant muscle is then stimulated electrically, however, it will immediately be able to start tapping again. What this experiment demonstrates is that it is not the muscle that has tired (since it is still responsive), nor is it the neuromotor nerve that has tired (since it is still capable of transmitting the necessary stimulus). What has tired is the gap between the nerve and the muscle—the synapse—which has ceased to transmit the nerve-to-muscle stimulus.

The lesson to be learnt from this experiment is that so-called muscle fatigue may not always be due to the tiring of the muscles themselves. It is of course true that muscles tire owing to an accumulation of lactic acid, arising as one effect of the temporary lack of oxygen, but certain kinds of fatigue which affect the muscles may in fact have their location in another part of the total muscle system. They may, as we have just observed, be connected with synapse failure; equally, the release of catecholamine (the stress hormone) into the blood during intense exercise can lead to a state of chronic fatigue sometimes associated with the 'overtraining syndrome'.

Since the treatment of any physiological problem depends on correct diagnosis, it is vital that we be alert to the multiplicity of factors which can contribute to the impairment of muscle performance if we are to take appropriate remedial action. In the case of muscle fatigue, for example, the problem can be one of nervous exhaustion leading to early synapse failure; in this case the need will be for rest or less frequent training—not so much to let the muscles recover as to provide more adequate rest-periods for the nervous system. The excessive release of catecholamine, on the other hand, will require less intensive and stressful training sessions rather than longer periods of rest. Again, fatigue due to lactic acid build-up requires simply that we pause briefly in our routine to allow it to subside.

The above example is but one illustration of the importance of a holistic approach to the human organism when considering the effect of exercise. In this context, it should be noted that the factors involved may not necessarily be those directly related to the exercise itself, but may be connected with the more general state of fitness and efficiency of operation of the body as a whole. A persistent problem for some trainers, for example, is a lack of weight gain (in the form of muscle gain) resulting from their workout regime. The most common response to this phenomenon is to put it down to the training method being used. It is certainly true that training methods can be a critical factor—and at times *the* critical factor—in the development of muscle size, but they are not by any means the sole factor. Merely piling more weight on the barbell (in the belief that a high-weight low-rep program will produce the desired gain) may well be totally misguided especially if the basic problem lies elsewhere.

It may be, for example, that the protein intake is insufficient, with the result that the muscles are not being 'fed' at a rate commensurate with their output during exercise; if this is the case, the body will not be able to make good during rest-periods the protein loss arising from the breakdown of muscle cells during training. Equally, the shortage may lie

in the carbohydrate area, with the result that the body is either converting its protein intake not into amino acids but into urea (eliminated
from the body in urine), or is not building up a supply of glycogen
(stored carbohydrate) in the muscles with the result that the body has to
use up the available protein instead. Where the problem is not one of
food intake, it may easily be in the timing of workouts; if these take
place too soon after a substantial meal, the demands made on the blood
supply by the digestive process will limit the amount of blood available
to the muscles and their responsiveness to exercise will in turn be
diminished. In all of these cases, the answer to the problem is to be
found not in the muscles themselves and the mechanics of their operation, but in the support systems whose maintenance and enhancement
are critical to muscular development. Once again, the answer lies not in
considering the muscles as an isolated phenomenon, but in recognising
that they are part of a much larger system the understanding of which
requires us to address the human organism as a whole.

In the following sections of this book, our aim will be to follow
through the implications of the holistic view of the exercising body
which we have been advocating here. In Part II we consider the main
factors involved in maximising the effect of exercise for optimum
muscular development: these may be thought of as the 'non-exercise'
factors involved in muscle-building which we see as integral to a holistic
regime which exploits the individual's full muscular potential. In Part
III we discuss the chief modes of exercise for strength and fitness
training and show how the Matrix Principle, embodying the tenets of
holistic weight training, combines the most advantageous features of
conventional exercise modes in a series of programs which provide each
body-part with a total workout of unparalleled effectiveness.

Part II

Holistic exercise—the training environment

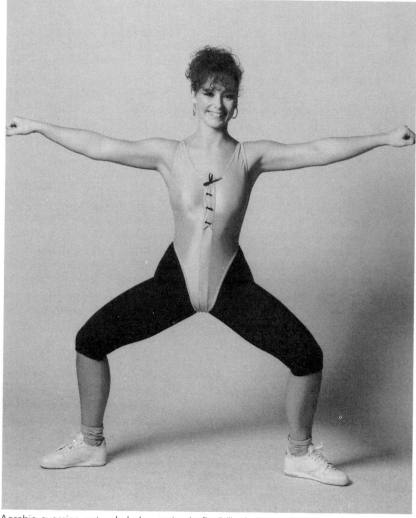

Aerobic exercise not only helps maintain flexibility but can also assist in speeding up the body's metabolic processes.

6 Exercise and health

It is more and more widely recognised nowadays that appropriate exercise can help us live healthier and longer lives. Although this exercise–health connection is sometimes dismissed as a popular myth, actuarial studies by insurance companies in the United States have indicated so significant a correlation between the two factors that one of the largest US insurance firms discounts by up to 35 per cent the annual premium on life insurance in cases where the policy-holders engage in recognised exercise programs of thirty or more minutes, three times a week. For those willing to exercise for at least one hour per session, five times a week, the reduction on life insurance premiums is even greater.

In the holistic context to which Part II of this book is devoted, two questions need to be answered at the outset. The first relates to the basis of the connection mentioned above: what is it about exercise that makes it so significant a factor in the maintenance and promotion of health? The second relates to the particular role played by weight training as a form of exercise. In this chapter, therefore, we shall explore the main dimensions of these issues.

Firstly, although the causal links are complex, at least one appears to lie in the genetic messages which have been imprinted in the human body over countless generations. In the earliest ages of human history not only did primitive people have to hunt to survive, but to survive they had to avoid being hunted. Savage beasts provided a source of food for them, but they also provided a source of food for those animals. Much time was thus taken up hunting and gathering, or avoiding being hunted and gathered. In such adverse conditions there is no doubt that exercise played a crucial role in the life of primitive humans. In short, they did a lot of running, walking and fighting; indeed they were constantly fighting for their lives.

Our biological inheritance thereby incorporated exercise or intense physical activity in the service of survival, and some of these survival mechanisms such as the 'fright take flight' kind still dominate our fundamental and instinctive responses. Our contemporary and more sedate, if not sedentary lifestyle, however, no longer provides an outlet for the physical activity which has been such an integral part of our socio-cultural evolution. The cholesterol problem we now face in health terms can at least be partly explained by this change in lifestyle. It has been suggested, for example, that the release of cholesterol in the bloodstream was functional when, with primitive weapons, our ancestors were hunting large animals. Given the likelihood that the animal would be wounded but not initially killed, the hunter would have to follow the animal until it dropped and this could have involved the hunter having to walk or run for literally days on end without food or rest.

In today's society, high-pressured jobs give rise to anxiety and stress which seem similarly to stimulate the release of cholesterol into the bloodstream but without the concomitant expenditure of physical energy which would in primitive times have utilised the cholesterol available. Whether or not this theory about cholesterol is accepted, it should be clear that because of our sedentary lifestyle we are generally getting less exercise than our evolutionary development over the course of nearly a million years has led our bodies to expect.

But what is the expectation of the body in physiological terms? What happens physiologically when we exercise? Exercise physiology is an enormously complex subject area, and we can restrict ourselves to an examination of only a few of the basic physiological aspects of exercise with a view to indicating the effect of weight training on these health-related factors.

Inasmuch as exercise affects the heart, it in turn affects the whole circulatory system and thus in some way impacts upon all of the seventy-five trillion cells in the body. Let us first consider how exercise does affect the heart. Put simply, the function of the heart is to pump blood, thereby supplying oxygen and nutrients to the cells while removing their waste products. On average the resting heart rate for adult males is about 70 beats per minute; for women between 75 and 80 beats per minute. The heart is itself a muscle, and with sensible exercise the heart muscle grows stronger and becomes a more effective pump. As the strength of the contraction is improved, stroke volume is increased, thus decreasing the number of beats per minute required for the heart to pump the same volume of blood. In consequence, the heart is no longer working as hard to do its job. Since every heart beat is a muscle contraction, the only chance the heart gets to rest is between beats. The stronger the heart, then, the more chance it gets to rest. Not only will the beat of the heart muscle remain lower at rest, it will also rise more slowly and work less hard to accommodate the blood supply demands of vigorous physical activity.

How, then, does exercise serve to improve cardiovascular fitness? We have already observed that the heart beat elevates during exercise to deliver a sufficient supply of blood to the specific muscle-groups which require more oxygen because of the processes described in Chapter 2.

The requirement for more oxygen stimulates breathing, thus allowing the lungs to supply the blood with more oxygen. During this process the tidal flow of air per minute (the inhalation–exhalation cycle) is increased from about six litres of air at rest to more than 45 litres during intense exercise. The lungs may be called upon to oxygenate the blood by more than 20 times its normal resting requirement.

During vigorous exercise the demand for additional oxygen is met by breathing faster and more deeply. These ventilation modifications are for the most part controlled by the involuntary reflex centre in the medulla responsible for respiration. This brain centre contains neurons which during inhalation stimulate contractions of the external intercostal muscles (between the ribs) and the muscle of the diaphragm. During exhalation other neurons activate the internal intercostals and diaphragm, thereby completing the oscillating character of the breathing process. Stretch receptors in the lungs monitor the cyclic changes of volume in the thoracic cavity and assist in governing the actual rate of oscillation. The level of carbon dioxide in arterial blood is perhaps the single most important factor in the remarkable co-ordination of the respiratory impulses, as the rate of breathing increases proportionally to the concentration of carbon dioxide in the blood.

The above discussion serves to highlight the role of vigorous exercise in promoting cardiovascular fitness. Some form of cardiovascular disease affects nearly 50 million Americans or about one-sixth of the

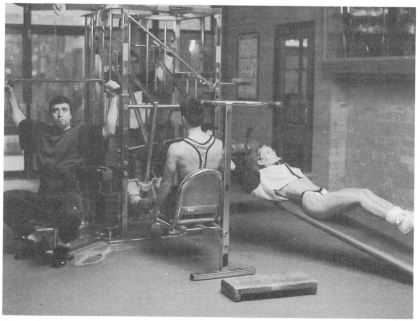

Circuit training is a form of vigorous weight exercise which helps promote cardiovascular fitness.

population, and Australia fares little better in percentage terms. Approximately 95 per cent of all heart attacks result from hardening of the arteries. The importance of this to our present subject is that it is now established that particular circuit-types of weight training can significantly benefit the cardiorespiratory system.

In 1986 researchers at the Oregon Health Sciences University in the US showed that with a group of previously untrained men and women, weight training over a period of four months brought about a reduction of 16.5 per cent in LDL cholesterol (low-density lipoprotein cholesterol), a significant factor in hardening of the arteries. In the same study, it was also shown that weight training caused an increase of 6.5 per cent in the levels of HDL (high-density lipoprotein cholesterol), which actually reduces the chances of atherosclerosis, thus assisting in the prevention of heart attacks.

In addition to the prevention of heart attack, exercise is now known to lower death rates in respect of a variety of other diseases. Again in the US, in a recent study undertaken by Dr Ralph Paffenburger et al. at Stanford University, it has been demonstrated that of 17 000 men, aged between 35 and 74 years, death rates were one-quarter to one-half lower in those whose weekly exercise regime expended at least 2000 calories. Death rates were further reduced by those whose caloric expenditure through exercise was around 3500.

There is some evidence to suggest also that nerve centres in the joints—stimulated by exercise such as weight training—signal the relevant centre of the brain responsible for breathing, muscular co-ordination and even bone regeneration. In addition to supporting the body, muscles move bones closer to each other through the process of contraction. As muscles grow stronger, the force they exert on bones through contraction is also greater. This being so, more calcium is deposited in the bones to make them strong enough to accommodate the increased force of muscle contraction. This is why exercise is so important in the rehabilitation process of broken bones and other skeletal deformation.

When bodily processes respond to exercise by making the kind of cardiovascular, skeletal and neuro-muscular changes to which we have been alluding, the process is called the training effect. Different exercises stimulate different training effects. The principle of specific adaptation to imposed demands (SAID) states that these different training effects can be physiologically classified. Aerobic exercise, for example, brings about a specific adaptation, being particularly well-suited to improve cardiovascular fitness, endurance, and flexibility. The word 'aerobic' means *with air* and refers to moderate intensity and sustained exercise which requires the body to use large but not intolerably large quantities of oxygen.

Because the quantity of oxygen demanded by the muscle cells is not overwhelming, aerobic exercise can be performed for protracted periods, thus making the heart grow stronger, improving the capacity of the lungs to process more air with less effort, and increasing the blood supply to the muscles. Aerobic activity not only stimulates a specific cardiovascular adaptation, it also speeds up metabolism during the exercise session and for several hours subsequently, thereby assisting weight reduction by ensuring that calories taken into the body are more readily burned.

Although weight trainers and bodybuilders often use aerobic exercise to assist in defining muscle, they know it will not in itself build muscle. Muscle building is a specific adaptation of a different kind, being effected by means of progressive resistance. The physiological mechanism involved in progressive resistance was outlined in Chapter 2, where we discussed the overload principle by which demands are placed on the muscle to which it is not accustomed; these demands force adaptive changes in size, shape and strength components of the muscle according to the particular *type* of demand made on it. Muscle cells have a complex adaptive physiology and no one m... can realise all possible adaptations. Particu... contraction, or 'pumping', are more effectiv... those demands on cell components which... Although different from aerobic exercise in t... tations it favours, vigorous weight training sh... a significant effect on the metabolic proces... important role in connection with a number... such as the reduction of excess weight.

[handwritten: BMR now = ideal; 3260 1800; 326 180; 3586 1980]

To overcome weight problems we need to understand the extent to which metabolism determines weight and thus the extent to which weight problems can be influenced by changing metabolism. A person's basic metabolic rate (referred to as BMR) indicates the amount of energy or kilojoules used in the maintenance of the physiological processes involved in such basic activities as walking, eating, breathing, sleeping and even digestion. You can calculate your BMR in a rough way by multiplying your weight (in pounds) by ten and then adding your weight (in pounds) to the total. As an example, assume that your weight is 140 lb (63.6 kg). Multiply 140 × 10 which equals 1400, and then add 140 to that total, thus giving you a BMR of 1540. 1540 refers to the number of calories per day you require to sustain these basic physiological processes (1 calorie = approx. 4.19 kilojoules). On the assumption that your physical activity is minimal, eating more than 1540 calories (6452 kilojoules) will cause an increase in weight and eating less than that number of calories will cause a decrease in weight.

This is, of course, only a rough guide. A number of studies, for example, have shown that some overweight people eat no more food than leaner people. The difference lies partly in the fact that overweight people almost invariably have slower metabolisms than lean people, thus increasing the time during which food is converted into body tissue. It is also the case that the sustenance of muscle requires energy expenditure even at rest, whereas fat does not: two people could weigh the same, for example, but if one of the two has a greater amount of lean bodyweight or muscle than the other, then that person will have a higher BMR than the other and will require a greater kilojoule intake. The more muscle we have, the more kilojoules we burn in maintaining that muscle. The greater the proportion of fat to muscle, the fewer kilojoules we need to sustain the fat; thus the lower BMR.

As with aerobic exercise, vigorous weight-training exercise temporarily increases the BMR for extended periods following a workout. After a vigorous weight workout, for example, your BMR could remain elevated for periods as long as eight hours. For those who like to eat, this means that they can eat more during the period of elevated BMR following the workout than before the workout while still preserving their overall balance of weight. Similarly, by controlling their appetite, exercisers can exploit the post-exercise BMR elevation period to assist them in losing weight. (This point will be explored in Chapter 9.)

Vigorous exercise contributes to the development of lean tissue and the minimisation of fatty tissue. By redressing the balance in favour of lean tissue, we alter the BMR so as to burn more kilojoules on a permanent basis even in an inactive state. A recent theory suggests that exercise causes an increase in the production of certain hormones which assist in the emulsification or breakdown of fat into free fatty acids which are used directly as a source of energy in muscle-building.

Given the correlation between obesity and a number of diseases, it is clear that weight control is an integral component in the prevention of disease and maintenance of good health. While dietary intake is of course an important factor in the control of weight, a controlled diet coupled with a regular exercise program will be not only more effective because of the post-exercise BMR effect, but by converting the kilojoule intake into muscle it tends to speed up metabolic processes and thus to have a more permanent effect than dieting alone.

7 The importance of lifestyle

Exercise is only one of a number of factors which contribute to overall health: it cannot be fully effective if the other aspects of our lives are not equally directed towards the achievement and maintenance of the ends which exercise is meant to serve. A holistic view of human well-being incorporates exercise into a total lifestyle whose other elements complement and enhance the benefits of exercise rather than (as can often happen) neutralising or even negating them.

The greater awareness in contemporary society of the value of weight training and other forms of exercise can present health educators with a dilemma. It is no doubt true that they will find a certain satisfaction in the fitness boom, as measured by the increases in gym enrolments and aerobic classes over the last decade. On the other hand, they often cannot escape a nagging reservation that disturbs any complacency they might otherwise have had in thinking that we have truly come to appreciate in health terms the value which exercise can have.

The commercialism of the fitness industry of course is itself a worry, but the reservation of health educators betrays a deeper concern based on the realisation that exercise is for many *not* being undertaken in the name of health. On the contrary, a number of people misuse exercise to perpetuate the unhealthy lifestyle to which it was hoped exercise might provide an alternative. Every day, responsible weight instructors bear witness to people who train diligently, yet either before the workout or after its completion, fill themselves with junk foods and animal fats, imbibe excessive quantities of alcohol, smoke cigarettes, and take even more harmful drugs. It is discouraging to find the benefits of exercise being reduced to a prophylactic against the continuous toxic assault which some weight trainers wittingly inflict upon themselves.

We noted in the previous chapter that exercise can be used legitimately to control weight. If the weight ideal to which one aspires is healthy, then the use of exercise to achieve that ideal can also be healthy. On the other hand, if the physical ideal to which one aspires is inimical

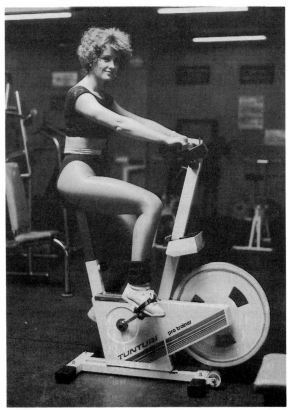

Healthy exercise in moderate amounts can help keep the body trim and attractive without resort to extreme measures based on an obsessive concern for weight reduction.

to or undermining of health, the use of exercise to achieve that ideal can be equally unhealthy.

One increasingly common example of the misuse of exercise arises in relation to people who exhibit eating disorders and use exercise to realise a physical goal or to sustain an eating habit which is by its very nature unhealthy. A particular form of this disorder, which tends to affect women weight trainers and aerobics trainers especially, is *anorexia nervosa* or aversion to food. Given that the average mature female sustains 25 per cent body fat (compared to 15 per cent in mature males), the preponderance of anorexia nervosa in women is understandable, given a simplistic view which equates the presence of excessive fat (and thus of *all* body fat) with an unsightly or unhealthy body. Anorexia is not a disease in the conventional sense of a degenerative physical process, but rather an obsessive syndrome based on a distorted self-image. It is characteristic of the anorexic's mentality that no matter how thin one is, one can and should be always thinner. Paradoxically, the subconscious ideal of the anorexic is the state of death, the condition in which, reduced to skin and bone, the human system no longer functions.

In this regard the use the anorexic makes of exercise is in the service of self-destruction, not of health.

Another example of conflict within the total working system can be seen in the cigarette-smoking exerciser. For some people, this habit is adopted or continued in the belief that it will prevent them from feeling hungry and that, by replacing food as a source of oral gratification, it will help keep their weight down. A number of bodybuilders have in recent years come to rely upon cigarette smoking as a normal part of their pre-contest preparation. The basic premise is that smoking assists in curbing appetite and increasing the free fatty acid of the blood, thus helping to rid the body of any excess fat.

The dangers of cigarette smoking are well documented, and while it is medically associated with lung and throat cancer, the incidence of deaths from heart disease among smokers is so astoundingly high that this risk factor alone should eliminate smoking from any lifestyle aimed at the pursuit of health. When cigarette smoking is coupled with the severe dietary regime to which bodybuilders and supposed 'health fanatics' submit themselves, the effects are greatly magnified. Oxygen deprivation and an accelerated thrombotic or clotting tendency are particularly evident and at their worst can lead to blackouts, fatal strokes, and even cardiac arrest. In its own way cigarette smoking can be as dangerous a practice for the bodybuilder or fitness trainer as the use of anabolic steroids.

Numerous other examples could be given of attempts to combine health-enhancing and health-destroying practices. Common to them all is an impaired sense of self-esteem. The scenario of the anorexic is importantly different from the case of those persons who refrain from eating too much or from eating too much of the wrong things because they wish to preserve or enhance the esteem in which they already hold themselves. Those who knowingly impair their lungs and hearts through cigarette smoking betray through their actions that they believe themselves to be no more worthy than the toxins they inhale. Holistic exercise trainers do not see the body as separable from the self; they genuinely want to improve their body because they value it as they value themselves. They are not trying to trade in their body for another model as though it were somehow disposable.

One of the most distressing examples of this syndrome of misuse, and unfortunately best-known in the world of weight training and bodybuilding, is that of the drug-taker. Just as some anorexics can never be thin enough, some athletes can never be strong enough or big enough, no matter how strong or big they are. Exercise becomes a means to an end, and so does the body. The health of the body is then sacrificed for the 'good of the cause', whatever the cause might be. If drugs serve the cause, then so much the better. Those doctors who have treated the users of anabolic steroids often have frightening stories to tell about bodybuilders who present with irreparable liver and kidney disorders, serious heart impairment and a variety of other symptoms, but who blithely dismiss the fact that they are pushing themselves towards an early grave with a comment such as (to quote an actual case in point): 'Yes, but I put an extra inch on my arms.' When the self-image being sought has degenerated to the degree where it negates the very purpose of our activity then something must be seriously wrong with the values held.

We have stressed the negative behavioural patterns which can have a powerful role in undermining the beneficial effect of an exercise regime. It is important, however, to stress equally the effect that exercise can have in enhancing the general well-being of the human organism when it is undertaken holistically; that is, as part of a total way of life aimed at maximising the healthy functioning of the body within its environment.

A significant example is to be found in relation to the incidence of certain viral diseases. Recent research has revealed that socio-cultural factors such as stress, alienation, environmental pollutants, and even the ingestion of some processed foods, can serve to depress the immune system, thereby making us vulnerable to diseases against which we would normally be protected. Chemicals such as phorbol esters (found in paint and paint thinners, wood strippers and also in furniture and floor polish) have been shown in laboratory conditions to depress the immune system sufficiently to permit the reactivation of viruses such as herpes which would otherwise be latent.

It is clear that patterns of disease, and more particularly those which have come to be called diseases of modern civilisation, cannot be understood independently of patterns of lifestyle. While stress is known to impair immune function, recent studies have shown that relaxation training through meditation elevates the blood levels of the thymus-derived T-cells which are responsible for the production of the disease-fighting anti-bodies destroyed by AIDS.

Other studies confirm the beneficial role which exercise can play in strengthening the immune system. During strenuous weight workouts, for example, the production by the brain of natural pain-killers called endorphins is known to improve the function of the immune system by enhancing the activity of a range of cells directly involved in the fight against disease. Research has also shown that exercise can increase the production of T-cells by stimulating the growth of the thymus gland. The thymus gland, located under the breastbone, monitors the conscription from the bloodstream of lymphocytes which are then programmed to function as T-cells. Similarly, studies reveal that exercise significantly augments the activity of interferon, another chemical naturally produced by the body in the fight against viruses and diseases.

There is also recent evidence to suggest that the elevation of body temperature that occurs in exercise such as weight training serves to enhance the capacity of the immune system to destroy viral invaders. Some studies even claim to show that exercise can influence the systemic functions of the body in such a way that the immune-effects of vitamins such as A and C are determinately bolstered.

Finally, it has been suggested that exercise can also contribute to mental well-being. Although the physiological connections between exercise and depression are not entirely clear, a considerable literature has accumulated on the benefits of exercise for stress management and associated forms of depression. Dr Rod Dishman of the University of California reports one recent Norwegian study, for example, in which a group of patients suffering from clinical depression responded more positively to psychotherapy when it was accompanied by regular exercise sessions. One theory proposes that vigorous exercise increases the amount of noradrenaline, a hormone which is known to affect moods, by four to six times. Coupled with increased levels of endorphin production in the brain during exercise, it is likely that feelings of well-being and mood elevation could be further enhanced, assuming the relative absence of other, and adverse, lifestyle factors.

The above considerations serve to bring into focus the interrelatedness of factors contributing to holistic health and well-being. Exercise is an important element in this total matrix, but it can be misconceived and misguided if not related to other health-related activities and to positive attitudinal factors. The 'exercise high' just described, for example, will be of negative rather than positive value if it merely reinforces a distorted self-image which treats the body's appearance as an end in itself: an object or commodity to be made bigger, stronger, thinner and so on, irrespective of the longer-term implications for the human person as a whole. On the other hand, if the body is understood as an integral part of the total self, and its functioning valued as part of the respect we hold for ourselves as human beings, then its physical development through exercise, like the development of a good singing voice or of mathematical or linguistic ability, becomes a healthy and productive form of the realisation of our full human potential.

Our discussion highlights the shortcomings of a purely mechanistic view of physical health and fitness. Sometimes referred to as 'healthism', this philosophy is based on the narrowly reductionist assumption that 'exercise' equals 'fitness' equals 'health'. If the body is viewed purely as a machine, independent of factors including the enjoyment of life and a positive attitude towards it, then simplistic dogmas such as 'fat is bad, thin is good', 'exercise makes you healthy' and the like, tend to be accepted in ways which can ultimately defeat the very ends they seek to promote. Exercise can indeed lead to fitness, and fitness can in turn foster physical health, but it is only when our concept of health embraces the well-being of the total person as a matrix of physical, emotional, attitudinal and social factors that fitness becomes a truly meaningful concept and the role of exercise in promoting it falls naturally and positively into place.

8   Weight training and age

A commonly accepted view of weight training is that it is of benefit only to adults, from the late teens to the age of about 35 to 40 years. We would argue, on the contrary, that although muscle growth may be most dramatic in the years of early adulthood, the practice of weight exercise as part of a holistic approach to fitness and health can also be beneficial well outside the age parameters mentioned above. The present chapter discusses the ways in which appropriate forms of weight training can be effectively used by both children and older adults to improve muscularity and to promote general fitness.

Children

The claim is often made that weight training is not good for children. Before offering a response to this claim, it is worth recalling that only a few years ago people were asking whether weight training was good for women, and not too long before that whether weight training was good for anyone. There is now no question that weight training is good for men, and it is also manifestly clear that it is of great benefit to women; this being so, why should it not be good for children as well?

The straightforward answer is that weight training can benefit any individual, young or old, healthy enough to engage in it, but there are some myths to dispel and some words of caution. The most widespread myth about the ill-effect of weights on children is that before the onset of puberty, lifting stunts the growth of children. This is a medically naive statement from a number of points of view. First, if weight training were a height depressant, reaching the onset of puberty before commencing training would hardly guarantee that the height of an individual would not subsequently be impaired. Since considerable growth takes place during the years following puberty, one could only safely commence weight training when full height potential had been reached. This would mean that some individuals should not even begin weight training until their early twenties; the great Steve Reeves (who began training in his teens) would not have even been a contender in the national titles that he won when in his early twenties.

The charge that weight training stunts children's height rests upon a spurious understanding of the physiology of growth. It derives from the notion that weightlifting fuses the epiphyses or soft growth plates at bone ends. (These are the points at which the bone is capable of extending itself, and fusing of the epiphyses refers to the closing or calcification of the connective tissue which provides the medium for bone growth.) Studies have demonstrated the opposite, however, and shown that appropriate weight-training programs can significantly improve skeletal and muscular patterns of growth in children. It is well known, for example, that Soviet weightlifters begin training between the ages of 11 and 13. In a study undertaken by L. S. Dvorkin in 1987 the training effects on weight-trained Russian children were monitored over a 15-year period. He concluded that as a result of prepubescent weight training, the subjects showed significant increases in muscular bodyweight and bone density not experienced by their non-weightlifting peers.

Other studies have shown that exercise itself stimulates the production of testosterone, the hormone primarily responsible for the development of male sex characteristics and muscle growth. While testosterone can directly affect the rate at which the epiphyses fuse, the increased production of testosterone as a consequence of the body's natural response to exercise does not serve to stunt growth. The reason for this is that the elevation in testosterone production brought about by exercise speeds up the process of total body growth, including height, at the same time as it speeds up the process by which the epiphyses come to be fused. Increased growth is thus proportional to the rate of epiphyseal calcification. The overall result, in terms of body height, is essentially the same. The difference is that exercise tends to increase the rate at which height and muscular growth are attained for both males and females. During the puberty phase, weight-trained males in particular seem on average to grow faster, become stronger and gain muscular bodyweight more rapidly than their peers.

Although the bones of prepubescent and adolescent children are flexible, undue and continual stress upon young bones can, however, cause a condition called Avascular Necrosis in which the blood supply to the epiphyseal plates is inhibited. The lack of appropriate blood supply leads in turn to a bone deformation known as Osteochondritis Disseccans in which the actual process of cell fusion essential to bone growth is impaired. Excessive stress upon the epiphyseal plate can also lead to other types of bone deformation such as slipped femoral epiphysis. Such conditions as these do provoke skeletal abnormalities and stunt growth. There is, however, no evidence to suggest that weight training produces sufficient stress upon bones to bring about these deleterious effects.

At the other end of the exercise versus bone-growth spectrum is the example of what were called the Battle of Britain children—children who during the Second World War were obliged to spend long hours in underground air shelters. Lack of sufficient exercise, coupled with lack of sunlight and inadequate diet, brought about a range of bone disorders but inhibited bone growth was predominant.

Our own research and personal experience indicates that children can begin to profit from weight training from the age of six onwards. Proper supervision is of course essential, and a child should no more be allowed to lift weights unsupervised than be allowed to swim in a pool unsupervised. The supervisor should be knowledgeable and understand the principles involved in lifting and how these principles apply to young children.

Before the child lifts weights the major emphasis should be on ensuring that the child achieves a basic state of general conditioning. Calisthenics, such as chin-ups (assisted as necessary), push-ups and dips, coupled with aerobic exercise, assist in increasing the overall level of fitness and strength. These exercises can later serve as a warm-up routine prior to an actual weight-training session. Light weights should be used to begin, ensuring that the child lifts and breathes properly; if the unloaded bar is too heavy, a broom stick or length of metal pipe will suffice until the movements are natural to the child. As the child becomes accustomed to the exercise regime, the weight can be gradually increased. Heavy lifting should be avoided, particularly lifting tied to exercises which are compressive. Light presses and light squats carefully monitored can, on the other hand, be beneficial in improving the body's respiratory and cardiovascular responses, while stretching exercises such as chin-ups and pullovers are extremely helpful in achieving skeletal transformations, as are cross-over cable exercises.

Finally, keeping an accurate record of height, weight and measurements, along with a photo album, can do wonders for morale, while providing objective assessments of progress. Children should train because they feel for themselves the benefits of weight training, not because they are told it will be good for them; in consequence, it is important to remember that just as men and women can train well together, so can families. There is much to be gained from the mutual encouragement given when family members are brought together in a shared activity.

Older adults

It would be unrealistic to deny that certain aspects of the ageing process diminish the prospects of a vital and healthy life. For one thing, lean muscle mass tends to decrease while bodyweight fat increases. The two are not unrelated, since lean bodyweight or muscle burns up kilojoules even when the muscles are at rest; unmobilised or metabolically inert fat cells, on the other hand, show no kilojoule-burning disposition. The decrease in lean bodyweight normally associated with the age of about 50 can result in a person's gaining 5 kg (11 lb) of fat in a year without having changed dietary habits or kilojoule intake, the fat increase result-

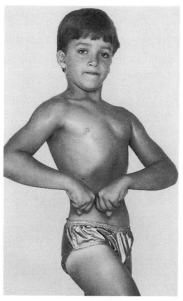

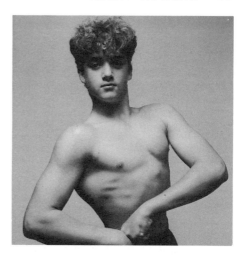

Adam Laura began weight training at the age of 6 under careful supervision by his father, Professor Ron Laura. At the age of 7, he was already showing impressive results (*left*) and at age 13 is outstandingly well developed (*above*).

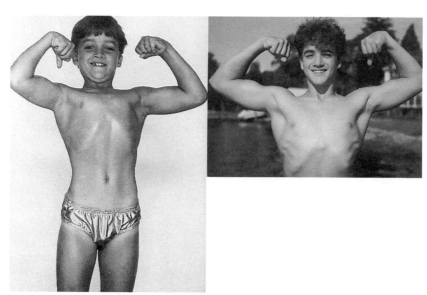

Contrary to some theories, weight training in early childhood does not inhibit the body's later development, as Adam Laura demonstrates. At the age of 13—height 185 cm (6 ft 1 in) and weight 80 kg (12 stone 8 lb)—he shows the increased muscular growth fostered by sensible weight training in childhood.

ing from a change in the internal metabolic process rather than from the amount of food intake. The fat increase of 5 kg is the result of the body reducing its daily kilojoule requirement by a mere 419 kilojoules (100 calories). The fatter we become, the more prone we become to degenerative diseases such as diabetes and heart disease.

Those individuals whose metabolism does not predispose them towards growing fatter in middle and old age will still have to contend with other factors. The more sedentary we become, the less fit we become, and the more difficult it is to reverse or even retard the ageing process. Along with losses in skin elasticity, ageing entails the decline of strength, co-ordination, testosterone production in males and females (thus affecting muscle density and muscle tone) and memory function. Skeletal disorders such as osteoarthrosis figure prominently, as do dysfunctions of the spine. The declining ability of the body to assimilate minerals such as zinc and chromium is less obvious, but like the degeneration of the thyroid contributes significantly to the signs and symptoms of ageing which *are* obvious.

Cellular changes associated with ageing are in fact evident in every organ of the body, though the rate of degeneration varies considerably. This suggests that certain muscles are more susceptible to the degeneration associated with the ageing process than are others. There is a body of evidence which indicates that the flexor muscles of the lower extremity and the extraocular muscles, for example, display degenerative patterns at a relatively early age. More specifically, it is thought that the force production of the quadriceps femoris muscle in the thigh is

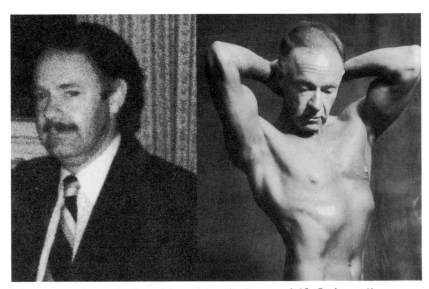

It is never too late to begin weight training. At the age of 40, Professor Ken Dutton was decidedly overweight and suffering from severe hypertension (*left*). At age 52, he has replaced his excess fat with lean muscle (*right*) and maintains his blood pressure well within the normal range.

predisposed as a function of age to degenerate both isokinetically and isometrically.

In the light of such a depressing picture, the question arises whether it is possible to do anything about the degeneration associated with ageing. The answer is in the affirmative, but its explanation points to the fact that what we can do to get 'out of the rocking chair' is precisely that which should keep us out of the rocking chair in the first place.

The first step in retarding the ageing process is overcoming the sedentariness which adversely affects the body's general health. In this regard exercise can play an important role, but it will apply differently to different people, depending upon whether they are presently sedentary or not. We need to distinguish between those individuals who currently exercise but who might otherwise be inclined to stop as they grow older, and those who are currently sedentary, having either undertaken vigorous exercise only in their earlier years or never having done so.

For those who currently exercise it is crucial to continue doing so if the ill-effects of old age are to be avoided: we are all aware of the severe atrophy or rapid wasting of muscle which follows the casting of a broken arm or other limb. Once we pass 30 years of age, atrophy of muscle due to inactivity is less acute but is nonetheless significant. The deterioration of muscle begins within 24 hours of immobilisation, and within a year of no systematic exercise the physiological advantage of the elite athlete over people who have never undertaken systematic exercise will have dissipated by at least 50 per cent. The message for those who do train is therefore to continue training regularly, but as they approach and pass middle age to train vigorously with lighter weights.

For every decade past the age of 30, the capacity of the heart to pump blood decreases in the average person by 6–8 per cent. However, in a recent study by Dr George Sheehan reported in the journal *Physician and Sports Medicine* (1986), a comparison was made between master athletes (aged 53–65) and untrained middle-aged men, on the one hand, and trained younger athletes on the other. The master athletes demonstrated oxygen uptakes 20 to 30 per cent higher than the untrained group and showed a decrease of only 5 per cent per decade (almost half the average decline exhibited by men over 25) when compared to the younger group. Based on a comparison with former champion runners who had ceased training for at least twenty years, the masters group demonstrated oxygen uptakes of more than 50 per cent in excess of those attained by the former champions.

It is clear, then, that from both muscular and cardiovascular points of view continuation of one's training into middle and older age can significantly retard the normal processes of ageing. The common misconception that as we grow older we need to exercise less should therefore be replaced by the understanding that in fact we need to exercise more.

In terms of muscular development, it is instructive to consider those who stand at the pinnacle of this process, namely professional body

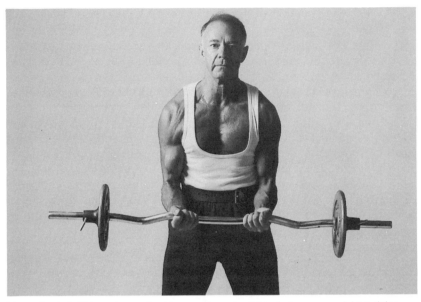

Those in their fifties who maintain a regular schedule of vigorous weight training can significantly delay the body's ageing processes.

builders. There was a time when it was unusual to see a bodybuilder past 40 years old in a professional bodybuilding competition: they tended to be restricted to the 'Masters' categories in amateur contests. Now the Olympia and other professional contests are filled, in open competition, with superstars in their forties. One of the best examples of a body-builder who has successfully held back the hands of time is Albert Beckles who, when in his mid-fifties, was defeating professional body-builders half his age. Other names that come to mind are those of Sergio Oliva, Frank Zane, Bill Pearl, Reg Park, Chris Dickerson, Boyer Coe, Johnny Fuller, Ed Corney, Larry Scott and Dennis Tinerino.

The training message is by no means confined to those who have exercised in their earlier years. Even in those of advanced age who have never undertaken serious training, the use of light weights in a regular exercise regime can produce beneficial effects ranging from enhanced cardiovascular fitness and endurance to increased flexibility, better toned muscles and skin, and improved general health. In addition to these purely physical consequences, the psychological outcomes they encourage are of vital importance: as the body begins to improve its overall fitness, so mental attitudes tend to become more positive and exercisers begin to 'think younger'. Slipping into frailty and infirmity can be as much a psychological symptom of old age as a physical one, so that the chief impediment to fostering a vigorous and active old age through weight training may well be the mistaken belief that one is already too old to begin.

Amongst the experimental subjects studied in the training clinics in which evaluation of the Matrix Principle has taken place over the past decade were a number of deliberately included older exercisers. One of the most striking of these subjects was a man 81 years of age who had never previously undertaken weight training. Since the system is based on the use of relatively light weights, we wished to test our hypothesis that it could be adapted to increase the strength levels of those in their seventies or eighties. The subject in question began the shoulder routine using a broom stick in place of the barbell. Having increased his original strength level many times over, he was able to move to the barbell, and at age 83 not only takes pride in his physical prowess but reports an increasing enjoyment of his enhanced mobility and a more active interest in the world around him.

The key to approaching Matrix training in later years is to warm up thoroughly and to select weights which are easy for the trainer to lift. Exercisers should concentrate initially on adopting the correct form and take the program gradually: at the outset, they should not feel obliged to complete the full stage of training indicated in the routines given in Part IV, but rather try to complete only one sequence in the stage, or perhaps only a couple of exercises in the sequence. We stress that the Matrix Principle is essentially a training *method*, not a rigid set of exercises to be performed slavishly by all exercisers regardless of age or physical condition. For most exercisers who take the time to adapt their bodies to the Matrix system, it will soon be possible to undertake the whole of Stage I without difficulty. Those who, because of age or infirmity, cannot follow the system even to this extent should not give up altogether: by concentrating on maintaining the exercise level that they *can* achieve, they are already taking an important step in counteracting the old age syndrome.

Part of the problem of old age, in fact, is that we live in a society which equates the natural ageing process with growing old and weak. We live in a society that celebrates youth, often at the expense of those persons who no longer possess it. Such a society creates the impression that the old retire because they are worn out and useless. The tragedy is that having come to believe this falsehood we transform it into a self-fulfilling prophecy, robbing ourselves of the lives we might otherwise have had. A holistic approach to weight training will take a very different attitude to the process of growing old: not one which takes refuge in fanciful notions of eternal youth or denies the natural cycle of the human organism, but rather one which refuses to accept that the effects of ageing should be encouraged and even hastened when it is possible to maintain a high measure of physical and mental vigour well into the later years of our lifespan.

9   The Matrix diet

The old adage 'You are what you eat' is nowhere more true than in the context of muscle building. We can exercise hard and often, even employ the most sophisticated muscle-building techniques known, but unless we fuel our bodies properly, our days of hard labour in the gym will be useless. Basically, we can only get out of our bodies what we put in.

The growing awareness amongst the athletic community of the fundamental importance of diet to sporting success and especially to the building of muscular strength is reflected in the abundant literature that has emerged in recent years. The shelves of bookstores are laden with works aimed at revealing the seemingly endless secrets of diet and nutrition, and it seems that no monthly lifestyle or health-oriented magazine would be complete without at least one article devoted to the topic. Our purpose in this chapter is not to summarise or even distil the myriad works already written on the subject, but to consider it from a somewhat different angle.

Along with the development of Matrix training has come a new level of understanding of the ways in which this type of exercise can be combined with dietary intake to promote maximum growth or maximum weight loss. The establishment of these relationships has been a by-product of the development and testing of the Matrix Principle, and as such represents a new approach to the diet/exercise connection.

Metabolism and weight

The reason there is no single kilojoule formula for weight gain or loss is that individual metabolisms differ. What is optimal for one person in regard to food intake may simply be inadequate for another. Metabolism is thus critical to the determination of how much muscle you can gain and how quickly you can gain it. Metabolism refers to the whole range of chemical and physiological processes by means of which a living organism produces energy to maintain its vital functions, including the replacement of cells, recuperation and muscle development.

Within the body, two aspects of the metabolic process dominate: the anabolic or building-up process and the catabolic or breaking-down process. Muscle building depends largely upon creating a positive anabolic state. The fundamental reason some people gain weight quickly and others gain it slowly is that the *rate* or speed at which these processes take place within the body varies considerably.

We noted in Chapter 6 that building muscle is itself a way of influencing metabolism, as is allowing ourselves to grow fat. It so happens that it takes more energy for a living organism to maintain the vital functions associated with a muscular body than a fat one. Indeed, there is evidence to show that while the sustenance of muscle cells requires considerable energy, the sustenance of fat cells requires virtually none. The fatter we are, then, the less energy we need to maintain our body-state, and the more muscular we are, the more energy we will require in order to maintain it, even when we are sedentary.

The Matrix Principle, metabolism and weight reduction

Although the exact physiological mechanisms by which the above changes take place are not entirely clear, the evidence accumulated over a decade of clinical testing suggests that Matrix training significantly affects metabolic rates. This phenomenon would explain why Matrix training can improve muscular definition at the same time as it increases muscular weight. The weight losses associated with Matrix *reduction* training indicate that the exercise regime stimulates metabolism and keeps it elevated not merely for several hours after the workout (as is the case with some conventional high-intensity workouts) but literally for days. Otherwise slow-moving, lethargic, overweight subjects using the Matrix system not only reported significantly greater weight losses than the control subjects in the conventional training group, but consistently expressed and exhibited heightened feelings of energy and vitality.

Subjects using Matrix training for weight reduction focused upon the bigger muscle-group exercises such as the leg, chest and shoulder Matrix routines and used those in conjunction with the dietary program later described. Clinical studies indicated that the greatest losses in waist measurement occurred amongst the Matrix control group in which no specific abdominal training took place in the first seven weeks of the program. There are several possible explanations for this. One hypothesis is that 'weight transference' or 'energy store transfer' (our preferred term) was facilitated by allowing the area from which weight was to be transferred to remain exercise-dormant. Another possible explanation is that because the abdominal muscles in fat people are generally underdeveloped, the immediate introduction of abdominal exercise makes the stomach muscles grow larger, with a minimal loss of the subcutaneous fat which covers them. This process would obviously inhibit the mechanisms by which the waist measurement is significantly reduced as a result of Matrix training.

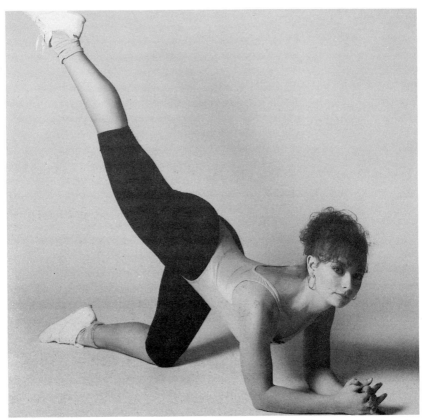

The maintenance of a lithe and flexible body can be assisted by a combination of a vigorous exercise regime and appropriate diet.

The Matrix weight reduction diet

There are various diets for weight loss which complement the metabolic effects of Matrix training. It should be remembered that one of the key characteristics of the Matrix Principle is *diversity*. Matrix dieting should also encourage diversity amongst the food sources which are incorporated into the diet regimen. The trainer, therefore, should not hesitate to substitute similar low-fat protein foods for the specific ones listed here. The table provided at the end of this chapter is meant as a helpful resource for selecting the most readily available low-fat substitutes in the diet set out below. It should be noted that butter, cheese and whole milk are eliminated from this diet. As with any diet, you should consult your medical practitioner before commencement.

Diet

Breakfast: soft-boiled or poached egg, 1 slice of wholemeal bread, 1 slice of pineapple and 1 glass of water or herbal tea (no milk or sugar).

Mid-morning snack: 1 piece of fresh fruit and a glass of pure fruit juice (freshly squeezed if possible).

Lunch: Baked, broiled or steamed fish with herbs and lemon, 1 baked potato, salad of lettuce, tomatoes, cucumbers, radishes, carrots, etc. (no dressing except for herbs and lemon).

Mid-afternoon snack: 1 piece of fresh fruit and a glass of pure fruit juice (freshly squeezed if possible).

Dinner: Tuna, salmon or chicken salad, a portion of melon such as cantaloupe, brown rice and vegetables (lightly steamed); 1 glass of water.

(Note that the tuna and salmon, if not fresh, should be packed in unsalted water, not oil. The chicken should be skinned before cooking.)

One of the major problems in maintaining a strict diet is control of hunger. Once the chemistry of hunger is learnt, however, the trainer can exorcise the demon of hunger and make dieting as easy as a walk in the park. Here are a few tips which should assist in mastering your appetite:

Eat sufficient fibre

As fibre passes through the digestive system, it absorbs water and swells, creating a sensation of fullness which allows you to limit your intake yet feel satisfied. Foods rich in fibre include bran, vegetables, fruits, cereals and whole grains.

Eat a little food more often

Your body burns kilojoules more efficiently if meals are smaller and more frequent as long breaks between meals cause your blood sugar to drop and your hunger to grow. Many people lose weight by eating five to six small but healthy snacks each day, taking the last snack of the day at least six hours before retiring.

Eat main meals in your most active hours

There are two peak energy periods which characterise the human system: mid-morning and late-afternoon. If you can't eat several small snacks during the day, try to confine your major food intake to just before your morning and late afternoon peaks, as your body will burn more kilojoules at these times.

Drink plenty of water

If you feel peckish between meals, drink water instead of eating. Water, occasionally accompanied by a piece of fruit which swells with the water, will decrease your hunger. A glass or two of water just before meals will also diminish your appetite.

Exercise

Few people ever maintain significant losses of weight without exercise. Exercise not only burns up kilojoules as you work, but speeds up your metabolism so that you continue to burn those kilojoules for a few hours after your exercise session. If you can't get to a gym for a vigorous workout, try a brisk walk which will make you feel less hungry and pleasantly refreshed.

Visualise your fat loss

The power of the mind in the control of hunger is critical. Take time on a couple of occasions throughout the day to relax and close your eyes to visualise your body as you would like it to be. Alternatively, picture yourself beginning an aerobic session. As the session proceeds, you see yourself getting firmer and fitter until you look the way you think you should. When you feel on the verge of a binge, combine some of the above techniques with a visualisation session to increase your inner strength and lower your appetite. Remember, you are not only what you eat; you are what you think.   → Pray. !!

Matrix diet for weight gain

Most athletes are interested in adding to their muscular bodyweight in order to increase strength and muscle size. Once again, the issue of metabolism deserves consideration, but this time from a different point of view. High metabolisms provide a special problem for those who wish to gain weight, since their bodies seem to require enormous quantities of food simply in order to maintain equilibrium. Since high-intensity exercise elevates metabolism, it may well be asked how any training, including Matrix training, could help to produce the rapid gains in muscle size which are claimed for it. The answer is relatively simple: it is extremely difficult to elevate the metabolism of a person whose metabolism is already elevated just as it is difficult to lower the metabolism of a person whose metabolism is already extremely low.

   The human organism works according to a principle called homeostasis. Homeostasis means that the organism will respond to demands upon it in a way that minimises the energy required for the body to do the job required; in other words, it is the way in which the body preserves its natural equilibrium. When a person's metabolism is already very high, any disposition to elevate it further is extremely disruptive of the equilibrium the homeostatic principle is meant to preserve. This being so, the body will tend to resist any further elevations of metabolism which would throw it further out of balance.

There will come a point at which the body will react homeostatically to a prolonged deprivation of kilojoules by maximising the efficient utilisation of the kilojoules from the food which is already available. The body protects itself from destruction, as it were, by introducing physiological mechanisms which dispose the human organism towards a return to equilibrium. High-intensity exercise, especially Matrix training, encourages the body to bring into play its natural disposition towards equilibrium. Should the metabolism already be high, for instance, Matrix training will encourage the slowing of the metabolism in order that the body can accommodate the increased demands with the minimum degree of disruption to the harmony of the system. This means that Matrix training can help even the slowest of gainers put on substantial muscle size when the training program is combined with appropriate diet.

Protein loading

With the exception of the water component of our bodies, protein represents about 20 per cent of total bodyweight and is the primary non-water constituent which makes up skeletal muscles. It is estimated that every six months there is a total renewal of the cells which compose our muscles. This constant process of cell replacement is hastened by high-intensity exercise, and though the issue has not been decided definitively, the weight of evidence seems to suggest that considerably more protein is required for muscle building than the conventional wisdom proposes. According to the recommended dietary allowances (RDA) established by the US National Academy of Sciences and the World Health Organisation, only 0.8 grams of protein per kilogram of bodyweight (1 gram = 0.002 lb) is required to sustain the body's daily requirements. Since nitrogen is a central component of protein, the interplay between protein production and protein breakdown in the body is measured by what are termed nitrogen balance studies. If the intake of nitrogen exceeds the amount of nitrogen excreted, a state of positive nitrogen balance exists and muscle growth is enhanced. Negative nitrogen balance occurs when nitrogen excretion exceeds the nitrogen intake.

Until recently, the orthodox view has been that muscle mass could not be increased if the body exhibited a negative nitrogen balance, and there has been widespread debate as to whether exercise alters protein metabolism sufficiently to hasten a nitrogen deficit. Our own clinical studies suggest that high-intensity exercise such as Matrix training decidedly increases the protein requirements of the athlete. This view is confirmed by Dr Scott Connelly who writes, 'any setting of an amount of protein theoretically necessary must be set against the background of activity (caloric requirements) . . . Without this, assigning someone an arbitrary daily protein need is ludicrous.' (S. Connelly, 'Just How Much Protein?', *Muscle and Fitness*, March 1990, pp. 101 ff.)

In addition, there are variations which arise from the digestibility of different types of protein. For example, egg protein is deemed to have an absorption factor of 97 per cent, whereas soybean protein exhibits an absorption factor of 90 per cent. If Matrix training does increase the level of daily protein requirement, and if sufficient protein is a major factor in the augmentation of muscle mass, how should one eat in order to achieve maximum growth? This brings us directly to the theory of protein loading.

The basic concept behind protein loading is that the homeostatic mechanisms which control the human organism's response to external stimuli will depend upon *the degree of disruption which a stimulus represents to the overall system*. There is a point at which too much protein will be regarded as threatening to the normal function of, say, the liver in metabolising protein. When this happens, the body eliminates the excess as faecal waste or stores it as fat. At the other end of the spectrum lies protein deprivation. Recent studies have shown that positive nitrogen balance is not a necessary condition of muscle growth. In experimental conditions, for example, increases in muscle mass have been observed in starving animals. The reason for this seemingly contradictory phenomenon is that at the point at which protein deprivation occurs, the body will protect itself so as to minimise the further dissolution of muscle mass by adjusting the efficiency ratios which govern the metabolism of protein. The amino acids which exist in different compartments of the body, for example, may be re-utilised to maximise the absorption of protein. The idea is not quite so foreign as it might at first seem. Cows, for instance, are known to chew their food, then regurgitate it after it has been partially digested in order to increase digestive efficiency. An even more peculiar but relevant example is that of the rabbit which will chew its own faecal matter in order to maximise the utilisation of any potential energy source.

Since Matrix exercise greatly increases the rate at which protein is broken down in the body, it follows that the daily recommended allowance of 0.8 grams for every kilogram of bodyweight is grossly inadequate. On the other hand, to increase at the outset of Matrix training the intake of protein to, say, 4 grams per kilogram of bodyweight would simply trigger the homeostatic mechanisms designed to eliminate the excess protein which may be disruptive to the metabolic equilibrium. One way of overcoming this problem is by *increasing protein intake by steps*, until a maximum efficiency point is reached, then peaked. At this point the protein intake is *reduced drastically* to trigger the homeostatic mechanism at the deprivation end of the spectrum. This obliges the body to compensate by increasing the efficiency ratio for the absorption of all its protein sources, including the re-utilisation of amino acids if necessary. The process of protein augmentation by steps to maximise the absorption of protein at every step is what we refer to as protein loading, a revolutionary concept which has proved itself in controlleld tests in Matrix training clinics. The traditional formula for protein intake recommends a *static* daily allowance, whereas protein loading recommends a carefully sequenced *variation* of daily allowance.

One example of a protein loading weight-gain diet for Matrix training is the following:

Week 1

Breakfast: 1 egg any style, wholemeal toast, cereal with fruit and whole milk.

Mid-morning snack: nuts (any kind), dried fruit and a milkshake.

Lunch: 1/4 chicken, potato (boiled, mashed or baked), vegetables, fresh fruit dessert, apple juice 1–2 glasses.

Mid-afternoon snack: tuna salad with wheat crackers or wholemeal bread, melon or fruit, freshly squeezed fruit juice, preferably pineapple.

Dinner: fish any style, rice (white or brown), vegetables, wholemeal bread and fruit dessert.

Week 2

Breakfast: 2 eggs any style, 1 slice of ham, wholemeal toast, cereal with fruit and whole milk, paw-paw or pineapple.

Mid-morning snack: chicken salad, melon and milkshake.

Lunch: fish any style, potato any style, vegetables, steamed, lightly boiled or stir-fried with onions and herbs. Apple juice 2–3 glasses.

Mid-afternoon snack: nuts, dried fruit, crackers and cheese, milkshake.

Dinner: roast lamb or beef (trim fat), vegetables any style, white or brown rice, wholemeal bread, fruit dessert, 2–3 glasses of apple juice.

Week 3

Breakfast: omelette with 3 eggs, toast, potatoes or rice and 2 slices of baked ham. Bran cereal of any kind with fresh fruit and whole milk. Paw-paw or pineapple, fruit juice.

Mid-morning snack: salmon or tuna sandwich with salad, nuts, dried fruit and a milkshake.

Lunch: turkey, chicken or duck, any style, vegetables, rice (white or brown), wholemeal bread, fruit cocktail dessert with ice cream (2 scoops), pineapple juice (preferably fresh).

Mid-afternoon snack: bean or lentil soup with pasta sprinkled with cheese, followed by a chicken salad sandwich and a milkshake with fruit and one lightly cooked soft-boiled egg.

Dinner: roast dinner of any kind with potato and vegetable, wholemeal bread, followed by fresh fruit dessert, pineapple slices, an apple or grape juice as a beverage.

Mid-evening snack: nuts, dried fruit, followed by a milkshake supplemented with a protein powder.

Week 4

Breakfast: omelette with 4 eggs, potatoes, cheese and three slices of baked ham. Bran cereal of any kind with fresh fruit and whole milk, paw-paw or pineapple, fresh fruit juice.

Mid-morning snack: 2 chicken salad sandwiches with salad, melon, nuts, dried fruit and 1 or 2 glasses of milkshake.

Lunch: spaghetti with meat sauce, meatloaf of minced lean beef or veal, vegetables and salad, wholemeal bread, dessert of crackers and cheese, fresh fruit, including fresh pineapple.

Mid-afternoon snack: pea soup with pieces of ham or a minestrone soup with pieces of chicken, nuts, dried fruit, followed by 1 or 2 glasses of a milkshake with one lightly boiled egg.

Dinner: fish any style, potato, vegetable, salad, wholemeal bread, fresh fruit dessert, crackers and cheese, and 1 to 3 glasses of fruit juice.

Mid-evening snack: 2 chicken salad sandwiches with salad, nuts, dried fruit, seeds such as pumpkin, 1 or 2 glasses of milkshake with fruit and 1 lightly boiled egg.

Once you have completed the fourth week of protein loading, your daily intake of protein should be around 4 grams per kilogram of bodyweight. It is now time to move from the point of maximum protein loading back to the minimum (or protein deprivation) level. Thus, in the fifth week, you repeat Week 1, in the sixth week, Week 2, and in the seventh week repeat the dietary regimen as in the third week, and so on.

The foregoing diet provides a balance of protein, carbohydrate and fats which, in combination with Matrix training, has been found highly effective in increasing muscular weight. The diet may be varied somewhat according to the appetite and preferences of individual trainers within the general principles explained above. A vegetarian diet high in protein could also be devised, but limitations of space require that the vast array of dietary possibilities be left to readers' ingenuity and common sense. As mentioned earlier, before commencing this or any diet you should check with your medical practitioner.

Table 1   Protein sources and percentage of protein absorbed and converted into muscle tissue

	Weight (grams)	Protein (grams)	Fat (grams)	Calories [1 cal = 4.1868 kJ]	Conversion rate (%)
EGGS					
Boiled or poached	100	13	11	158	88
Omelette	100	12	17	201	88
Scrambled	100	12	17	201	88
White	62	7	trace	32	88
Yolk	34	5	10	116	88
FISH					
Bass, baked	227	43	2.5	195	78
Cod, baked	227	38	1	370	78
Crabmeat, fresh, cooked	227	34	4	200	78
Fishsticks, frozen, breaded, cooked	227	36	20	400	78
Flounder, baked	227	36	1.5	158	78
Halibut, broiled with butter	227	44	2	194	78
Herring, kippered	200	38	10	242	78
Lobster, steamed	227	37	3	179	78
Oysters, raw	238	25	5	150	78
Perch, yellow, broiled	227	44	2	195	78
Red snapper, grilled	227	45	2	198	78
Salmon, canned	227	41	13	315	78
Salmon, fresh, broiled	227	43	14	298	78
Scallops, steamed	227	35	0.5	183	78
Shrimp, boiled or steamed	227	41	1.5	206	78

Table 1 (*continued*)

	Weight (grams)	Protein (grams)	Fat (grams)	Calories [1 cal = 4.1868 kJ]	Conversion rate (%)
Squid, poached, steamed	227	37	2	190	78
Trout, grilled	227	46	24	400	78
Tuna in oil	227	55	46	653	78
Tuna in water	227	63	1.5	288	78
MEATS					
Beef					
Hamburger, broiled, lean	227	35	22	338	68
regular	227	30	44	516	68
Round steak, lean, fried	227	45	27	423	68
T-bone, porterhouse, rib, sirloin steak, broiled	227	30	78	822	68
Lamb					
Chops, broiled	227	33	65	717	68
Leg, roasted	227	33	60	672	68
Pork					
Bacon, fried crisp or broiled	227	10	75	715	68
Chops, broiled	227	20	125	1205	68
Ham, smoked, baked	227	35	60	680	68
Roast	227	20	125	1205	68
Spareribs, braised	227	28	85	877	68
Veal					
Cutlet, broiled	227	40	43	547	68
Chops	227	40	45	565	68
Roast	227	40	43	547	68
POULTRY					
Chicken, dark meat, broiled	227	40	15	295	68
Chicken, white meat, broiled	227	40	14	286	68
Duck, roasted	227	36	65	738	68
Turkey, dark meat, roasted	227	44	10	266	68
Turkey, white meat, roasted	227	44	9	257	68

Table 1 (*continued*)

	Weight (g)	Protein (g)	Fat (g)	Carbo-hydrates (g)	Calories	Conversion rate (%)
CHEESE						
Blue	57	12	18	0	210	76
Cheddar	57	14	18	3	230	76
Cottage, creamed	227	31	9	8	242	76
Cottage, whole curd	227	38	1	8	193	76
Cream	85	7	32	4	322	76
Edam	57	13	15	1	195	76
Feta	57	8	12	1	144	76
Mozzarella (part skim)	57	13	9	1.5	139	76
Parmesan, grated	5	2	2	0	26	76
Ricotta (whole milk)	57	6.5	7	1	93	76
Ricotta (part skim)	57	6	4.5	3	77	76
Roquefort	57	12	17	1	205	76
Swiss	57	16	16	0	208	76
MILK AND CREAM						
Chocolate milk (1% fat)	244	8	2	10	90	76
Heavy cream	16	0.5	5.5	23	52	74
Milkshake						
chocolate, thick	344	11	18	58	421	74
vanilla, thick	344	13	11	61	387	74
Partly skimmed milk, 2% non-fat milk						
solids added	246	8	5	12	125	76
skimmed milk	245	8	1	12	89	76
sour cream	12	4	2.5	0.5	28	76
whole milk	244	8	9	11.5	159	76
Yogurt, no fruit made with						
skimmed milk	227	13	0.5	18	129	76
made with whole milk	227	8	7.5	11	146	76
Yogurt, no sugar with fruit						
whole milk	227	9	9	30	250	76
BREAD						
Commercial loaf	100	7	7	29	207	40
French or Italian	20	2	0.4	11	56	15
Rye	23	2	0.4	11	56	21
White, enriched	23	2	0.5	12	61	15
Whole wheat	23	3	0.4	10	56	21
CEREAL						
Bran flakes 40%	40	4	0.5	27	144	48
Cornflakes	25	2	trace	21	92	40
Oatmeal, cooked	236	5	2	23	130	48
Puffed wheat	14	1	0.5	12	57	48
Shredded wheat	28	4	0.5	20	101	48
Wheat germ	6	2	1	2	25	48
Wheat germ cereal cooked	65	20	8	25	252	48

Table 1 (*continued*)

	Weight (g)	Protein (g)	Fat (g)	Carbo-hydrates (g)	Calories	Conversion rate (%)
FLOUR FOODS AND RICE						
Macaroni and spaghetti cooked firm (8 to 10 minutes)	130	6	1	39	189	48
Noodles, egg, cooked tender (5 to 6 minutes)	160	7	2	38	198	48
Pancakes						
white flour	27	2	2	9	62	15
buckwheat flour	27	2	2	7	54	20
Pizza, small, white flour,						
cheese	75	9	6	24	186	60
sausage	100	8	12	23	232	60
Rice, brown	150	4	1	38	177	70
instant, white	147	3	trace	37	160	60
white	150	3	trace	36	156	63
FRUITS						
Apple	150	trace		18	110	
Apricots	114	1		14	55	
Avocado	215	5	33	11	361	48
Banana	151	2	trace	29	124	48
Cantaloupe	385	1		14	160	
Cherries	130	2		20	80	
Dates, pitted	175	4	1	115	485	48
Figs	114	1		23	90	
Grapefruit	285	1		14	55	
Grapes						
red	152	2	1.5	21	105	48
green, seedless	200	1	trace	24	100	48
Orange	180	2	0.5	18	85	48
Paw paw	400	2	0.5	35	152	48
Pear	180	1	1	24	70	48
Strawberries	150	1	0.5	12	57	48
Lemon	106	1		6	20	
Peach	114	1		10	35	
Pineapple, diced	140	1		19	75	
Plum	60	trace		7	25	
Tangerine	114	1		10	40	
Watermelon	925	2		27	115	
NUTS (shelled)						
Almonds, raw	140	26	75	2	785	35
Brazil, raw	300	42	201	2	1985	35
Cashews, roasted						
unsalted	100	15	45	26	569	35
Coconut, fresh	100	4	35	4	347	35
Unsalted peanuts,						
roasted	240	60	106	51	1398	35
Peanut butter	16	4	8	2	96	35
Pecans, raw, halves	104	10	74	6	730	35
Pistachios, roasted	100	19	53	10	593	35
Walnuts, raw, halves	100	21	60	1	628	35

Table 1 (*continued*)

	Weight (g)	Protein (g)	Fat (g)	Carbo-hydrates (g)	Calories	Conversion rate (%)
SEEDS (shelled)						
Pumpkin	230	67	106	12	1270	35
Sesame	230	42	122	18	1338	35
Sunflower	100	24	43	19	559	35
VEGETABLES (fresh)						
Asparagus, cooked	175	4		6	135	
Beans						
lima, cooked	170	13		32	189	
snap, green, cooked	125	2		7	30	
Beets, diced, cooked	165	2		12	50	
Broccoli, cooked	150	5		2	64	
Cabbage, cooked	170	2		7	35	
Carrots, sliced, cooked	145	1		10	45	
Cauliflower, flowerets,						
cooked	120	3		3	24	
Celery, raw	40	trace		2	5	
Corn, whole kernels						
from cob, cooked	200	4		27	133	
Cucumber, raw	207	1		7	30	
Lettuce, raw	220	3		6	30	
Onions, raw	110	2		10	40	
Peas, cooked	160	9		19	115	
Potato, baked	99	3		21	90	
Spinach, cooked	100	3		3	24	
Sprouts, bean, cooked	100	3		4	28	
Tomato, raw	150	7		2	35	
Yams, baked	110	2		36	155	

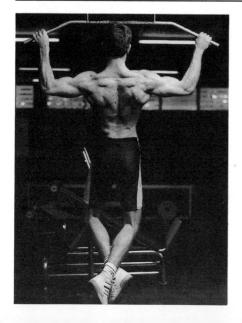

Muscle mass is significantly determined by the body's protein uptake.

10   Ergogenic aids

Whenever exercise has been undertaken for its own sake rather than as a corollary of physical labour or recreational activity, its practitioners have called on the assistance of external aids for the development of muscular strength or size. In ancient Greece, for example, athletes would often use a form of dumbbell (known as *halteres*) in their training in order to add to the momentum provided by the muscles in sports involving jumping or leaping. The physical culture movement of the 19th century, which began in Europe and spread to the USA with the waves of European immigrants, was quick to adopt Indian clubs and solid dumbbells as an aid to developing muscular fitness, and by the beginning of the 20th century these had been joined by the plate-loading adjustable barbell (invented in 1902) as well as by various patent mechanical devices and contraptions for which the most amazing claims were sometimes made. From the spring-loaded or rubber 'chest expanders' of

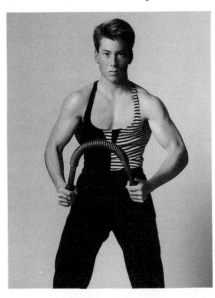

The 'power crusher' is one of many similar devices used to produce muscle resistance.

a couple of generations ago to the Bullworkers and 'flab-blasters' of more recent times, the search for readily marketable means of producing resistance to the action of the muscles has been unremitting.

Whilst the basic equipment of the muscle builder still remains the barbell and set of dumbbells, the latter part of the 20th century saw considerable advances in the application of mechanical theories of muscular action with the invention of training machines capable of exercising and isolating individual muscles or muscle-groups in highly effective ways. Standard circular weights were soon attached to various rigid frames to produce leg-press machines, Smith machines, calf-raise machines and the like, to supplement the standard array of 'free weights' and in the second half of the century such systems as Universal, Nautilus and Hydra-gym became a feature of better-equipped gymnasiums. Schools of thought soon arose as to the relative effectiveness of free-weight and machine training, though with the increasing sophistication of ergonomic technology the place of machines in weight training from the beginner's level to professional bodybuilding is now assured.

The most dramatic development in providing artificial means of assistance to muscular development was, however, to be of a chemical rather than a mechanical nature. The use of diet supplements, which had been a common feature of muscle-building regimes for half a century or more, raised few questions in terms of its appropriateness to health-oriented activities, but with the introduction of anabolic steroids, and their increasing use since the 1950s in certain sports requiring explosive muscle power, extremely complex issues surfaced. Bodybuilding, particularly at the advanced and professional levels, finds itself in the thick of these controversies. There is no need to recount at length the damage done to the image of healthy sporting competition, particularly at the Olympic level, by the use of performance-enhancing drugs; the well-publicised expulsions from the 1988 Olympics and other international athletic competitions indicate the extent to which sport has been robbed of its recreational purpose and become an instrument for furthering a self-serving form of national pride and financial ambition.

One misconception about the role played by drugs is that artificial aids aimed at improving athletic performance appeared on the sports scene only in the early 1950s in response to the desire of competitive bodybuilders and weightlifters for success in their respective sports. While this may be a reasonably accurate explanation for the introduction of synthetic anabolic steroids, it overlooks the fact that doping has been a pervasive part of sport for more than two millennia. At the Greek Olympics in the 3rd century BC competitors followed the lead of soldiers and later of gladiators in preparing themselves for their tasks by dining on hallucinogenic mushrooms, assorted seeds and herbal stimulants. By the mid-1800s athletes used ergogenics such as alcohol, caffeine, sugar-nitroglycerine, opium and even ethyl ether, all with an aim to improving their physical capabilities. By the turn of the 20th century the stimulant strychnine was added to the list and was later joined by

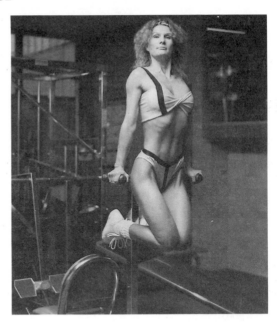

Vigorous exercise can be used to promote well-built and muscular bodies without recourse to potentially harmful artificial substances.

amphetamines, nicotinic acid and, more recently, anabolic steroids, testosterone injections, beta-blockers, diuretics and blood packing (the process whereby blood is removed from an athlete, frozen preserved for a period of several months and then returned to the athlete at the time of competition).

The current trend includes synthetic and genetically engineered forms of human growth hormone (HGH) and human chorionic gonadotropin (HCG). Although children suffering from hormonal deficiencies of a number of kinds have traditionally been treated with HGH, using HGH to increase size and strength in adults can produce a number of side-effects. One of the best known of these is acromegaly, a disorder of the pituitary associated with enlarged hands and feet, thickened lips and tongue, and facial distortions including a jutting lower jaw. The most commonly documented of the major adverse effects of steroids relate to liver dysfunction and the formation of liver tumours and liver cysts.

Other studies reveal a correlation between steroid consumption and testicular and prostate cancer. Steroids have also been linked to high blood pressure and increased cholesterol, both of which figure as significant risk factors in relation to heart disease. In addition, prolonged steroid use can lead to infertility, impotence, testicular atrophy, acne, baldness, pronounced female characteristics in men and, in women, male characteristics which include clitoral enlargement, cessation of menstruation and the lowering of the voice register. There is also literature accumulating which suggests that steroids are psychologically addictive. It is known they can be fatal: in Western countries alone it has been estimated that some 70 elite athletes have died in the post-war period as a consequence of doping.

The use of drugs is widespread: there is no one explanation, but there are many reasons; one has to do with the way in which our culture encourages our craving for instant satisfaction and for maximum achievement with minimum effort. 'Pill popping' is an example of this which is manifested within bodybuilding in the commercialisation of ergogenics. Not all ergogenics, of course, have the same medicinal status. Glandular extracts are natural food-based aids, whereas synthetic anabolic steroids are chemically based. People have come to rely more heavily upon chemical ergogenics because they believe them to be more effective in bringing about the physiological transformations they seek. Whilst there may be some evidence for the speed at which they work, there is also evidence to show that, in addition to the health risks involved, the quick gains made using synthetic steroids are counter-balanced by rapid losses upon the cessation of doping.

Another reason for the popularity of doping lies in the fact that many bodybuilders are under the illusion that it is possible, by means of drugs, to transform an immature body into the mature body of a champion without the hard work usually associated with the transformation. Less naively, other bodybuilders who have paid their dues in terms of hard work turn to drugs to overcome their sticking-points in respect of either size, strength, muscular definition or weight. More naively, others succumb to the pressures of competitive bodybuilding, to the glory of winning no matter what the cost, and to dreams of film stardom.

But what are anabolic steroids and how do they work? Anabolic steroids represent a particular group of steroids whose primary action is the stimulation of processes involved in the constructive phase of metabolism. Metabolism refers to the range of physiological processes through which the production, maintenance and degeneration of cell material take place. Metabolic processes divide into two main phases: the *anabolic* and the *catabolic*. Catabolism signifies the negative or destructive phase of metabolism in which complex substances are broken down into less complex materials. The positive or constructive phase of metabolism in which simple nutritive elements are converted into more complex ones is the anabolic phase. Those steroids with anabolic properties are called androgenic, a word deriving from the Greek meaning male-producing. Chemically-based anabolic steroids are synthesised on the model of the male sex hormone and contribute, as do natural androgens, to the anabolic phase by stimulating the body's production of cellular protein.

Of the body's androgenic hormones, testosterone is the most potent. The central production of testosterone occurs in the interstitial cells of the testes called the Leydig cells at a rate of synthesis of between 4 and 10 mg per day in males and approximately 0.1 mg per day in females. In the transition from the pre-pubescent to the pubescent stage in males, the production of testosterone increases 20-fold and muscle weight is increased 14-fold. Testosterone-induced changes in skin, distribution of hair, enlargement of the larynx, testes and associated sex glands are arbitrarily classified as androgenic effects, while testosterone-induced changes in blood, bone and muscle have become labelled as anabolic effects.

In the production of synthetic anabolic steroid, the structure of the testosterone molecule upon which it is modelled is manipulated so as to minimise the androgenic (or male sex characteristic) effects and to maximise the anabolic (or muscle-stimulating) effects. Unfortunately, the attempts to produce a purely anabolic steroid have not yet met with success. Two points are important to notice in this pursuit. First, the manipulation of the structure of the testosterone molecule increases the likelihood of imbalances in the body's assimilation patterns of the synthetic steroid. Nature has its own wisdom in ensuring that both the anabolic *and* androgenic effects of testosterone continue to occur. Its androgenic effects stimulate the accumulation of protein in advance of other tissues in the accessory sex glands, liver and kidneys, for example, so that the glands and organs which assist anabolic processes are themselves strengthened. This subtle process constitutes part of the body's internal mechanisms for the reception of the increased anabolic demands placed upon it. It would seem that the closer we come to the synthesisation of a purely anabolic steroid without the otherwise associated androgenic changes, the further we stray from ensuring the maintenance of the bodily processes capable of sustaining its anabolic effects.

The second point to be borne in mind is that the anabolic and androgenic effects of synthetic steroids are dependent upon factors other than the structure of the testosterone molecule itself. The duration of administration of the drug, diet, relevant dosages and the individual's level of testosterone-tolerance will all make a difference as to the dispersal of anabolic–androgenic effects. It is clear that even minor disruptions can adversely affect the body's control systems which regulate processes such as the rate of ageing.

The present discussion of anabolic steroids has been restricted to 'single-track' steroid administration; that is, to case studies in which only one type of hormone is used. It has been demonstrated that the difference between the strength increases shown by the anabolic and non-anabolic control groups amongst experienced weight-trained subjects cannot be explained purely as a placebo or psychological effect. In more recent case studies of steroid loading (i.e. combining different steroids, which are frequently taken in conjunction with testosterone) the increases in the anabolic test subjects have been even more dramatic. Unfortunately, the health risks associated with their combined administration are also dramatically increased.

The increasing incidence of the misuse and abuse of synthetic steroids is alarming and undermines the basic purpose of weight training to build strong and healthy bodies. The irony is that there are alternatives to the synthetic steroid syndrome, and that far too few sportspersons and weight trainers are aware of them. Whilst there is no alternative to hard work in building an outstanding body, there are natural ways of ensuring that the beneficial results of hard work are maximised. Turning away from synthetic steroids to food-based ergogenic aids and vitamin supplements is one effective approach.

Natural stimulation of the bodybuilder's endocrine system can safely be achieved through the use of currently available ergogenic nutritional aids. Glandular concentrates, for example, provide a way of maximising muscular growth by stimulating the endocrine system to produce naturally the same anabolic hormones that would otherwise be produced artificially by synthetic steroids.

Recent research on the anabolic effect of glandular-based aids demonstrates that they can benefit the bodybuilder in at least two ways. First, they supply ergogenic substances capable of activating the body's own production of androgens, whereas synthetic anabolics diminish the body's natural capacity for this production. While it used to be thought that the biologically active properties of glandular concentrates and other nutritional supplements are deactivated in the process of digestion, recent studies have shown that a sufficient portion of glandular extract survives to activate anabolically the body's hormonal functions. Second, glandular extracts, along with other health supplements, provide a rich source of high-quality protein without the fat content associated with the original foods from which they derive.

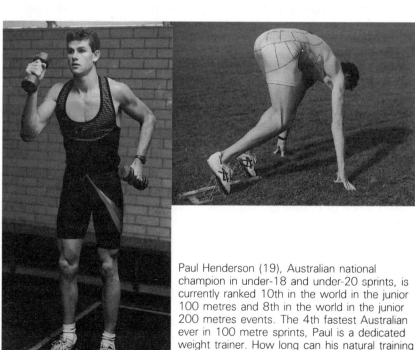

Paul Henderson (19), Australian national champion in under-18 and under-20 sprints, is currently ranked 10th in the world in the junior 100 metres and 8th in the world in the junior 200 metres events. The 4th fastest Australian ever in 100 metre sprints, Paul is a dedicated weight trainer. How long can his natural training methods hold out against artificial performance enhancement in world-class athletics?

The quest for artificial means of increasing athletic performance shows no sign of abating. Recent experiments involving the hormone erythropoietin (EPO) have been carried out at the Karolinska Institute in Stockholm, Sweden, with results so dramatic as to pose in acute form the problem of defining what may be regarded as natural, as distinct from artificially-induced, athletic ability. EPO is normally produced in minute amounts within the human kidney, its role being to stimulate bone-marrow to create oxygen-carrying red blood cells. Recent scientific advances have enabled the hormone to be artificially produced in the laboratory by bacteria implanted with the human gene that directs cells to make the substance. Administered in small doses, EPO can enhance the oxygen-carrying capacity of blood by some 33 per cent; the resulting increased circulatory capacity can in turn improve performance in aerobically-based sports such as running, cycling or swimming by an average of 10 per cent, thus providing athletes with a significant edge over their competitors.

Like the now outlawed practice of blood packing, EPO injection presents the problem that because the presence of the substance in the body is natural its artificial augmentation is practically undetectable. Since the differences in performance ability between elite athletes are considerably less than the boost provided by EPO administration, it has already been predicted by the world's foremost expert in this field, Professor Bjorn Ekblom, that its use could totally ruin athletic sport.

The holistic approach to physical performance that we have taken in this book is based on a value-system which places the realisation of our natural potentialities above the achievement of abnormal prowess by artificially-induced means. Natural diet supplementation is one way of improving physical ability without interference in the body's own chemistry or the harmful side-effects of drugs. But is is not the only way. In Part III of this book, we discuss the means of promoting muscle growth by natural, or drug-free, processes associated with the use of high-intensity exercise. The Matrix Principle is based upon the most recent research by exercise physiologists as to the forms of weight training most favourable to rapid muscle gain. By use of the Matrix training method, supplemented as appropriate by other forms of exercise, those who reject the 'quick fix' mentality of the drug-taker can, we believe, achieve similar levels of muscle growth by means of the body's natural response to exercise rather than by recourse to artificial and potentially lethal ergogenic aids.

11 Genetic engineering and the future

As we approach the 21st century, no account of the impact of techno-logical knowledge on the quest for muscular development would be complete without reference to the fascinating but disturbing possibilities offered by the technology of genetic engineering. Some of these possi-bilities, if realised, would render the contemporary debates concerning steroid use obsolete because of the immeasurably greater degree of physical control that could be effected. At the same time, they would produce (and are already producing) some of the most difficult dilem-mas ever faced by humanity in terms of its social, ethical and religious values. Space does not permit more than a cursory treatment here, but at least some of the issues to be faced will emerge from the following brief account.

Reference was made in Chapter 4 to the pioneering work of Watson and Crick who, in 1953, first analysed the structure of the genetic substance DNA, the carrier of genetic messages in the body. The next important advance in this field occurred in 1973, when researchers found that special enzymes could be used to cut a strand of DNA to which one could attach another strand of DNA taken from an entirely different person or living organism. Using the introduced DNA as a template or gene model, the DNA repaired itself by incorporating and replicating the new genetic material as a novel trait to be passed down from one generation to the next. This recombinant DNA technique is called gene splicing and it makes possible the altering of the genetic traits of one individual by introducing the relevant genes of another.

Although bodybuilders are familiar with the concept of increasing muscular size with the aid of growth hormone, the notion of genetically engineering such changes would, to most ears, sound like science fiction. If an appropriate source of growth hormone were genetically spliced into humans, it would literally re-program the whole growth pattern of an individual so that the resultant biochemical changes would be part of normal body function. There would be a single and uniform program of growth, and it would dictate the body's responses not only to exercise, but to a whole host of other physiological factors involved in muscular development. In the case of injected growth hormone, the body is obliged to cope with its own regulatory system plus the influence of the 'alien' growth hormone substances. In this case the introduction of an injected growth hormone works by upsetting the biochemistry and internal balance of the body, whereas gene splicing works by re-setting the body's biochemistry to bring about a new internal balance.

Gene splicing has momentous implications for the future of human-kind in general and the future of sporting performance in particular. We have for the first time in the history of the human race the power to shape our own evolution and to govern our own genetic potential. Genetic engineering would have the capacity to make anabolic steroids and other artificial ergogenic aids a thing of the past for, once the genetic disposition of a cell is altered, its subsequent processes take place as naturally as if it had not been altered.

During the past few years, progress has been made in building a computer designed to identify polypeptide sequences for molecules linked to specific genetic functions. The identification scheme provides for the isolation of some thousand or so specific gene locations. These locations form what is called a gene map which allows in principle for the manipulation of a wide range of genetically-induced characteristics such as skin pigmentation, male pattern baldness, height, shoulder width, hip structure, the length of the calves and perhaps even the rate of muscular growth. Utilising the recombinant DNA techniques of

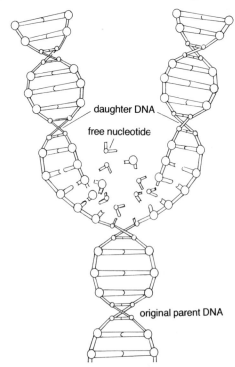

daughter DNA

free nucleotide

original parent DNA

A schematic representation of the DNA 'double helix' showing its capacity to split and thus replicate the body's genetic code

which we spoke earlier, it would be possibile to splice genetic material donated by an individual with a specific genetic trait (e.g. wide shoulders) on to the relevant DNA chain of another individual, thereby altering the recipient's shoulder width. It is in principle possible to combine the best physical traits of a number of top bodybuilders, thus producing a single individual who embodies them all. A human body could virtually be sculpted from the best genetic material the gene pool had to offer.

Still more complex issues are posed by the techniques available for cloning; for reproducing the exact genetic make-up of one individual in another. Given the already existing technology of embryo freezing, it now becomes theoretically possible to produce a replica of an older person. Imagine, for example that a number of clones are produced through engineered division of the original embryo and that the original embryo is implanted and brought to maturity, while the remaining clones are frozen. Several years might pass, providing sufficient time for the parents to assess its intellectual, physical and personality traits. On the assumption that the parents were satisfied, they could then choose to have a cloned embryo thawed, implanted and brought to maturity as a normal sibling would be. The main difference is that these siblings are identical twins, but born years apart. The process could be repeated and, in so doing, a couple could rear a family of clones. Indeed, the situation becomes even more remarkable when one considers that the embryos could in principle remain frozen indefinitely. This means that the original child could grow to adulthood, become a Mr or Ms Olympia, and then decide on one or more of the embryos in respect of which they are genetically identical. A Mr or Ms Olympia could thus choose to rear his or her own clone as his or her child. In the case of a Mr Olympia, the cloned embryo could be carried by his wife or a surrogate mother if necessary. In the case of a Ms Olympia, she could be made pregnant with her own clone. The permutations are mind-boggling. Imagine that our original child grew to adulthood, married and had children in the usual way (though a number of frozen clones could be utilised for this purpose). Imagine now that upon reaching adulthood the children of our original child decided to rear their father's clones. This would in effect mean that they would be rearing a genetically exact replica of their father, his clone, or their uncle, depending upon your feel for family relationships.

It is clear that the possibilities offered by genetic engineering would affect not only the building of bodies, but also the sport of competitive bodybuilding. To date, bodybuilding has been concerned predominantly with maximising genetic potential in respect of what might be called quality muscular growth. Ergogenic aids, including the use of anabolic steroids and other enhancement drugs, do little more than speed up and occasionally exaggerate the complex physiological processes by which food-protein is converted into muscle mass. While a bodybuilder may be able to increase significantly the size of his or her high calves, the genetic

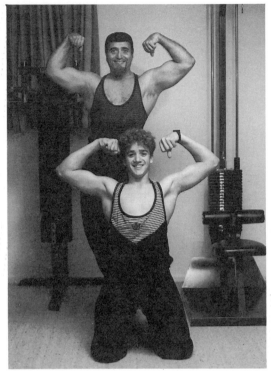

The genetic 'messages' that can sometimes be passed down from one generation to another are graphically illustrated in these photos of Prof. Ron Laura and his son Adam. Note in particular how Ron's wide shoulders and broad back have been inherited in Adam's genetic make-up. Modern genetic techniques such as gene splicing and cloning could enable such natural gene messages to be scientifically guaranteed.

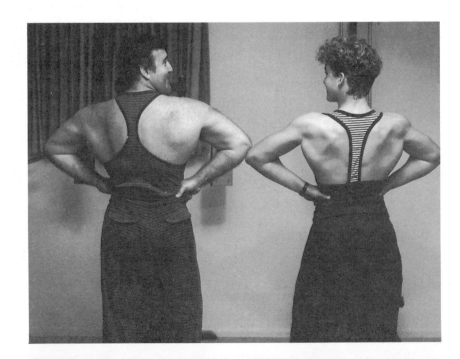

program of the individual will ultimately determine whether it is long or short calves whose growth potential is being maximised. The same principle applies to shoulder width, length of biceps, width of hips and so on. When all the hard training and dieting are done, it is basically genetics which will determine the law of successful outcome.

The direction in which research on human genetic engineering is currently being pursued has, it should be observed, led primarily to attempts to eliminate 'bad genes'. Given that 80 per cent of all babies born mentally retarded are victims of diseases of genetic origin, it is not surprising that considerable effort is being directed towards advancing this area of application. The transition from the aim of eliminating genetic defects to the goal of making genetic improvements such as the bodybuilder might seek amounts, in effect, to the way one views two sides of the same coin.

The concept of a 'defect' acquires its negative force when viewed as a condition we have no wish or need to tolerate. An IQ of 100, for example, would normally be considered acceptable, and an IQ lower than this tends to be seen, to a greater or lesser extent, as a defect. Suppose, however, that recombinant DNA procedures were used standardly to increase the IQ of most children to, say, 150. The previously acceptable IQ of 100 would come to be regarded as unacceptable—it would be seen as a defect.

The issue is not simply: If we are willing to eliminate 'bad genes', why should we be unwilling to improve upon 'good' ones? The issue is that genetic manipulation would by its very nature alter irrevocably the concept of 'good' and 'bad'. If we can genetically engineer 58 cm (23-inch) arms, have we not devalued a 48 cm or even a 50 cm arm gained through honest labour?

Were we supporters of genetic manipulation we could suggest that this problem would be overcome by democratising the genetic basis of competitive sport. To achieve this, we would ultimately engineer a hybrid athlete whose genetic character would reflect a range of preferred traits deriving from, say, the top ten bodybuilders in the Mr Olympia or Ms Olympia lineup. Then, using the hybrid as a genetic template, we could clone a pool of potential competitors, each of whom would have the same genetic chance of success as any other. If this were to happen, the standards of the competition would doubtless be extremely high but the contest would be boring. Part of what makes any competition exciting is that genetic variation provides for a kaleidoscope of diverse body-types. Needless to say, judging a lineup of bodybuilding clones would be a nightmare, We would be looking simply to determine how well the competitors realised the *same* genetic potential.

It may well be that genetic engineering will be used as the ultimate performance-boosting aid. If it can be established that no *harm* is done to an athlete in the process, what grounds would sporting organisations have to prohibit performance-boosting transformations? Perhaps it will be necessary to reinstate and reformulate the concept of fair play to set a standard against which an unfair competitive advantage could be judged.

Genetic engineering provokes a whole host of ethical considerations which require reflection and must be resolved by society in the very near future. It is not our purpose here to evaluate the moral propriety of genetic engineering, but simply to show that it is not a futuristic dream but a current possibility; not science fiction, but scientific fact. Should the techniques described above become generally available, there will without a shadow of doubt be many people who will wish to make use of them. The way in which we resolve these issues will make more of a difference than any of us might think to the kind of world (including the sporting world) in which perhaps we and certainly our posterity will live. In this case, the values of those who are committed to a holistic view of human development will be sorely tested, and they will need to decide whether we believe we possess the godlike wisdom to make decisions which can so irrevocably affect, and in such large measure determine, the lives of other human beings or whether our common humanity is better served by the development of the potential with which we are naturally endowed.

Part III

The weight-training workout

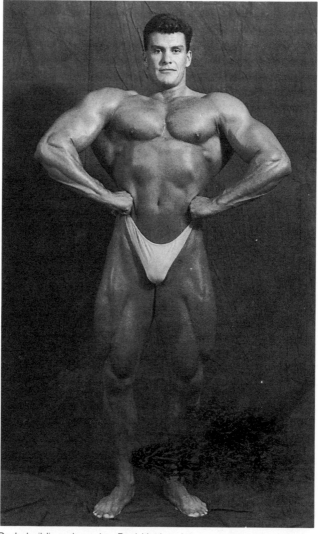

Body building champion Paul Haslam has an outstanding physique, the result of a naturally favourable genetic configuration refined and developed by years of intense training. Not every weight trainer can aspire to this degree of muscular development.

12 Training methods

One aspect of weight training which some trainers find totally fascinating is often experienced by others as little more than confusing, and even as a source of discouragement. We refer here to the multitude of training methods recommended in the many and various textbooks and articles devoted to the subject, not to mention the even greater variety of methods endorsed by well-known athletes and bodybuilders. It seems that, for every expert recommending (say) a high-intensity method with multiple sets of low weights, there will be another who will state categorically that only a heavy-weight workout with a maximum of three sets will produce substantial muscle gain.

It is entirely natural that, in a field of activity such as the quest for muscular development which, for some trainers, becomes an all-consuming passion and even an obsession, there will be a constant and never-ending search for the perfect training routine. Even top body-builders can sometimes be heard to complain that they are not yet satisfied with the look of their physique and are still searching for the elusive technique that will finally enable them to overcome their weaker points. More commonly, those trainers who are looking for a quick and easy solution to their problems and sticking-points will switch incessantly from one training method to another in the expectation that one of them will prove to be the missing key to a miraculous transformation. It is no wonder, against this background, that there is a large and receptive audience for any new method of training that comes along.

Equally, however, many weight trainers, especially those who have only recently started out and are looking for guidance, are frankly perplexed by the seemingly infinite number of techniques, routines and programs that they find prescribed, as they turn from one text or manual to another, or as they hear one instructor denigrate or dismiss the training method that another instructor has so confidently recommended. It may even seem to them that they are moving in a world of hypotheses and theories, and that none of the so-called experts or authorities really knows the answers to the questions asked. As with the first group of trainers mentioned above, the bookshelves of these learners are often filled with a variety of works on weight-training methods, each tried for a time and then, for many different reasons, abandoned in favour of some new method. One of the problems with textbooks (and even some instructors), for example, is that their prescriptions are often geared to practising or potential competitive bodybuilders, and thus do not cater for those trainers who either do not have such an ambition or whose weight training is meant as an adjunct and an aid to sports training.

In our view, the true situation in respect of weight training lies somewhat between the extremes mentioned above. On the one hand, there is no such thing as a 'miracle' training method, and the learner who has been led to believe that one particular method, to the exclusion of others, will bring about a sudden and startling process of muscular development where others have failed has been sadly misinformed. On the other hand, it must be recognised that because each method of training differs from others, each placing a different set of demands on the muscle system, there will be some which will be more effective than others in promoting muscle growth in certain learners whose muscular system responds well to the particular pattern of stress and overload imposed by a particular technique or set of techniques.

Our own approach takes heed of the particular genetic configuration we inherit at birth and its determining effect on the degree of muscular growth of which we are capable. The very mechanics of muscular action will impose limits on, for instance, the capacity of some people to lift heavy weights, because of such factors as the relative length of their bones or the points of insertion of individual muscles. The age and sex of the trainer, state of general health and other lifestyle factors, and even the stage of life at which training begins, can play a major part in the inherent capacity of that particular body to respond to the overload effect of weight training. Finally, individual bodily metabolisms can play an important role in regulating or restricting the conversion of our nutritional energy intake into mechanical energy production and the fostering of muscle growth.

Such factors should make us wary of any claim that a particular training system can fundamentally transform a physique. We should repeat here what we have said earlier: the most effective technique of growth-oriented weight training will aim at producing the maximum degree of muscle growth *of which that particular body is capable*, given the limiting factors mentioned above. Also, since different bodies respond in different ways, no single method of weight training will be ideally adapted to all trainers, and a certain amount of judicious experimentation may be necessary before the trainer can assess which method or methods suit him or her best.

We can summarise the above by saying that any recognised form of weight training can be effective, provided that it is performed correctly (i.e. in the right manner, with the required frequency, and for an appropriate length of time) and provided it is well adapted to the trainer's own physical constitution and realistic goals. What is all-important, and the main theme running through the first part of this book, is that trainers should *understand* what happens when they exercise with weights, so that they can use that information to find their own way through the myriad techniques, methods and routines that may be suggested to them, and discover which combinations are best adapted to their aspirations and potential.

We are therefore attempting, in the present section of this book, to concentrate not so much on introducing the entire range of exercises that can be performed and the various modes of performing them, but on the relation between *cause* and *effect* in the main types of exercise you will come across in your reading and personal instruction. Though some suggestions are made as to training routines which can be carried out in various modes, we stress that our aim is to encourage trainers to *understand* the effect of these different types of training, so that their own experimentation, or the reading of training manuals devoted to various exercise methods, may be built on a solid basis of information and not on the slavish following of either one set of instructions or another.

The final chapter in this section is devoted to a general discussion of the Matrix Principle, the particular method of weight training which this book introduces for the first time. It is important, however, to establish at the outset precisely what is, and is not, being claimed in relation to the Matrix mode of exercise.

Firstly, it is not being presented as some miracle system for the rapid transformation of puny weaklings into muscular marvels. To do so would run counter to everything we have said and would be totally misleading. For one thing, it is a form of high-intensity exercise which relies for its effect on the significant demands it makes on the muscle system. Although the earlier stages of each Matrix make some allowance for those who have not yet gained complete proficiency, it involves such a range and number of movements combined with very short pauses between sets that it simply cannot be performed in accordance with instructions without an intense concentration of muscular energy. The 'transformations' it produces will be the result of a period of disciplined, intense and demanding exercise which trains the muscles into new forms of adaptive response. There is nothing miraculous about this process, and whether or not the hyperplasia theory is accepted as a reason for its effect, the resultant gains are achieved only through determined training.

Secondly, and for the above reason, recuperation times are important between Matrix sessions, and it is therefore best seen as a form of ultra-efficient training to be backed up between sessions by conventional but less demanding modes of training. In this sense, it is part of a total exercise regime rather than a substitute for other forms of exercise. In the chapters which follow, therefore, we discuss the main forms of conventional weight training which may be appropriate for, and helpful to, exercisers at various stages of their physical development. Each of them, we believe, has its value (some for more advanced trainers, others for beginners and older exercisers), and each can be combined appropriately with Matrix training.

Finally, to return to a point made above, while our tests over a ten-year period have shown vastly more dramatic muscle gains through Matrix training than through any conventional training mode with which it has been compared in controlled tests, the natural limitations imposed by genetics, age and similar factors cannot be completely overcome by either the Matrix or any other training method. What can be claimed with confidence is that the Matrix training system has shown itself more capable than any other single weight-training technique of promoting the development of muscular growth. We therefore believe that it comes closer than any other natural training method to producing the maximum muscular development of which the individual trainer is capable. Clearly, the results obtained will depend on how far the trainer progresses with the Matrix routines—each seven-stage routine exists in introductory, intermediate and advanced forms—but even the introductory routines provided will, if properly followed, enable the trainer to make a significant degree of progress towards realising his or her full muscular potential.

13 Workout variety

A high percentage of those who have decided to embark on a program of weight training adopt one of the standard forms of training (sometimes known as training styles) and stick slavishly to it, month after month and year after year. There is, however, much to be said for the kind of program which either includes various types of exercise in the regular workout or switches from one to another at periodic intervals. Most of the standard weight-training exercises can readily be adapted to different training styles, and the trainer can often benefit markedly from exposure to as wide a variety as possible.

The main variations in workout style are brought about by:

- increasing its *intensity* (i.e. lifting the same total weight, but in less time);
- altering the *load* (i.e. using lighter or heavier weights);
- varying the *number* of sets (or of repetitions per set);
- changing the training *mode* (e.g. from isotonic to isometric exercise).

There is much benefit to be gained from a properly planned program which switches from one workout style to another. In the first place, a change in exercise style can help avoid the feeling of boredom or lack of motivation which sometimes affects exercisers. Those whose regular routine is unvaryingly the same not infrequently find, perhaps after some months or even in a shorter time, that they are no longer deriving the same 'buzz' from it that characterised their first discovery of the joys of weight training: the well-known 'exercise high' may start to prove elusive, and there may be a very real temptation at this stage to give up the practice of weights completely. The members' records in gymnasiums are often full of case-histories of those who had enrolled for a given period but abandoned the attempt before the period of their enrolment was over. While this is often due to unrealistic expectations (e.g. miraculous transformations arising from a minimum of exertion), a further well-known cause is the loss of enthusiasm arising from the repetition of exactly the same workout over an extended period of time.

A second reason for varying the workout style is that, while every recognised form of exercise brings its own benefits, it inevitably limits the trainer to those benefits alone and thereby restricts his or her access to the advantages offered by alternative forms. Each type of exercise brings into play an individual combination of physiological processes, but since the latter are of great complexity in their effect on the neuro-motor system, no single method of stimulating and exercising the system can aspire to completeness.

Thirdly, and perhaps most importantly, maximum muscle development requires us to call upon all the resources of the physical system of which the muscles are a part. We noted in Chapter 2 that the muscles operate in response to a set of signals generated by the brain and conveyed by the motor nerves. From the very earliest age, the body learns how to react to these signals and is soon able to respond in extremely sophisticated ways. The principle of energy conservation, however, means that in general the body will only respond to the signals we send it to the extent necessary to perform the required task. With time, the strenuous operation of the muscles through exercise renders them more adept at carrying out the demands our training makes upon them: the muscles grow, our metabolic processes transform our improved nutritional intake into more efficiently used motor energy, and exercises which at first we found difficult become noticeably easier. It not infrequently happens, however, that after an initial period of muscle growth we cease to make the kind of gains noticeable in our earlier training: we reach a plateau and assume that we have reached the maximum gain of which we are capable. Worse still, we may even find that we begin to lose a certain amount of the hard-won muscle growth that we noticed earlier. This is sometimes attributed to the phenomenon known as overtraining, and it is certainly true that if there is insufficient recuperation time between workouts this may well be an important factor. The real cause, however, could just as easily lie somewhere else.

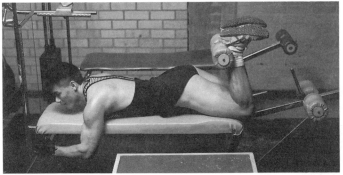

Some exercises, like the leg curl, are naturally painful, especially for beginners. Perseverance is needed in overcoming pain barriers and maintaining the challenge to the muscles to work harder.

Given that the muscular system has gained in efficiency in the early months of training, the principle of energy conservation to which we referred above will now come into play, so that the exercise which required considerable effort when training began may now require much less exertion. The muscles, in fact, have 'learnt' how to perform the movement against the resistance imposed, and from now on will perform it using the least necessary energy. As the required energy is now less than it was when training commenced, the demands on the muscle system diminish in consequence. The same exercise which, just a few months ago, required specific muscles to operate to their maximum capacity can now be performed with much less stress on these muscles than previously, and the latter will cease to grow and may even decrease in size as a response to the lower level of stress being placed on them. A standard response to this phenomenon is to increase the amount of weight lifted, but this process can be taken only so far until a point is reached where the weights simply become too heavy and the risk of strain and other injury increases.

Whilst it is important to increase weight levels beyond those used by beginners, and to maintain this form of mechanical challenge to the muscles at a level commensurate with the number of repetitions needed to pump the muscles and stimulate growth, this is far from being a complete answer to the problem described. What we are suggesting is that it is desirable, from time to time, to 'shock' the muscles by subjecting them to different types of exercise.

Set out in the next chapter are a number of different forms of exercise which can be combined with Matrix workouts to constitute a total weight-training program. For maximum muscle gain, it is strongly recommended that the trainer should have recourse to at least some if not all of them: in this way the muscle system will be exposed to a more complete range of tasks which exploits its potential. It is best if this process is not undertaken haphazardly, but rather according to a set schedule which ensures that each exercise mode is adequately utilised.

There are a number of ways in which this can be done. The following suggestions may be helpful, but it should be noted that they apply to those workouts (or parts of workouts) which are performed *other than by the Matrix method*. The Matrix Principle should be used according to the schedule given in Part IV, and the conventional exercise modes (as varied from time to time) can then be organised around it. Thus, each workout will consist of (a) a Matrix routine for a particular body-part, and (b) conventional routines for one or more other body-parts, performed in a style which the trainer can alter as set out below.

Our research indicates that trainers who prefer each workout to be in a single style will find that (assuming at least three or four workouts per week) a period of 8–10 weeks is desirable before switching to a different style. This gives the body time to adjust to the form of exercise selected and obtain the maximum gain from it before the next mode is undertaken and the muscles shocked into a new adaptation. For competitive bodybuilders or those aspiring to competition, the standard training style will consist of anaerobic isotonic training with relatively heavy weights, so that training in other modes will obviously be done for shorter periods. On the other hand, children and those who take up weight training in their later year will tailór the various modes so as to stress light-weight and isometric training.

There is no reason why a number of different exercise styles should not be combined in the one workout; for instance, at a given time the arms may be being exercised in low-weight, high-rep mode and the legs in high-weight, low-rep mode and so on. This adds variety to the workout, but the trainer should be careful to recall the schedules being followed for the various body-parts. To attempt to combine a number of different modes for the same body-part in the same workout can negate the shock effect which is produced by accustoming the muscles to one mode over several weeks and then switching to another mode, unless, of course, the combination is itself used for a short period as a shock method.

Whatever type of training is being undertaken, it is important that the appropriate mix of exercise and recuperation be adopted. What is 'appropriate' varies so much from one individual to another, depending on the age, stage of training, the type of exercise and individual metabolic rate, that any tendency towards dogmatism must be avoided in this matter even more than in others. Even top professional bodybuilders will differ markedly in their training routines and rest periods: some train for up to six hours every day, whereas others find that an hour or so five days a week is sufficient to keep them in top shape. To make this observation, however, ignores so many factors—the intensity of the workout (i.e. just how much is packed into a limited time with minimum breaks between sets), the particular body-parts worked on specific days and thus the recuperation time available for each—that its sole value is to indicate the variety of effective means of organising one's training.

A few general principles do, however, apply. In the first place, one or two workouts per week will generally be insufficient to keep the body at its best. To understand this, it is helpful to think in terms of the trainer as the teacher and the body as the learner: the body needs, in a metaphorical sense, to be taught that it is an *exercising* body; that is, that the 'norm' to which it is called on to conform is that of a regular output of significant muscular energy. To maintain the body basically in a state where no major muscular output is required, and then to subject it sporadically to bursts of muscle training, is unlikely to keep the body in a state of preparedness whereby the muscles retain a high degree of tone and build up an increasing capacity to cope with the regular demands being placed upon them. The gains made in one exercise session are dissipated well before the next session takes place. Moreover, the demands on the cardiovascular system made by occasional bursts of high activity may be severe (as witness the phenomenon of heart-attacks suffered on the squash court by players who try to mix a low general level of physical activity with occasional 'all-out' exercise), and the risk of muscle strain is also intensified by such kinds of training.

The most practical approach is to have a weekly schedule of exercise. Of the seven days available, we consider that at least four should contain a time-slot devoted to exercise. In this way, at least four out of seven days—a majority of the week—will be exercise days, and this means that the body is an exercising body on more days than it is a resting body. We are, in other words, teaching the body that exercise rather than non-exercise is the norm for its regular functioning. If the number of exercise days drops to three, the majority of days in each week become non-exercise days and the body will respond less effectively.

Crucial to this whole discussion, however, is the need for adequate recuperation. It is vital to remember that muscle is not built in the gym: it is built in the period following the gym workout, and in particular during sleep. What the gym workout does is *stress* muscle (a very different thing from straining it), requiring it to respond in a heightened way to the demands made on it. If the stress is not repeated within a given period, of course, the muscles will respond, according to the principle of energy conservation, by reverting to their former state.

What this indicates, then, is that although a recuperation period is necessary for muscular growth, this period must not be too long or the gains from exercise will again be lost. The recuperation period required will vary according to the amount of stress placed on the muscles during the exercise session, so that a high-stress workout (e.g. high weight or high intensity) will require a longer period than its low-stress counter-part. A muscle-group which is subjected to high stress will require up to four days' recuperation (depending to some extent on the general fitness of the trainer), since higher levels of fitness tend to shorten the recuperation time needed. Low-stress exercise, on the other hand, can be engaged in on a daily basis with only a good night's sleep being required for recuperation. Those who have acquired good muscle tone in the abdominal muscles can do several sets of sit-ups daily (using only their own body-weight for resistance) whereas, at the other extreme, a session devoted to 'blitzing' the arms or legs through a high intensity workout or heavy curls and squats will require three or four days' rest of the relevant muscles before they should be trained hard again.

This explains why advanced bodybuilders can, and often do, train daily; their workouts are so organised that each training session may concentrate on a particular body-part which is 'hit hard', sometimes to the point of exhaustion; this body-part will then not be subjected to high-stress exercise for the next few days which are devoted to other muscle-groups or to forms of exercise other than weight training (e.g. posing or aerobic training). It is in this sense that very advanced bodybuilders will sometimes state that their aim is to spend as little time in the gym as possible. Their weight workout is of such intensity that to prolong it beyond the point of maximum efficiency would incur the risk of overtraining and thus actually decrease the results they obtain. On the other hand, those who are training for general fitness will usually find that the lighter type of workout in which they engage will enable them to work each body-part thoroughly at three- or even two-day intervals.

Because the Matrix Principle requires that the muscle areas be intensely overloaded, the Matrix routine for any individual body-part should be performed only once or twice per week. It should be supplemented during the week by conventional training techniques, but these should be organised in such a way that the body-part exercised in Matrix mode is rested for three or four days before it is hit again in Matrix or conventional mode. Suggested Matrix schedules are provided in Part IV of this book.

With the above provisos, we recommend that for maximum overall fitness and muscle-tone, a weekly routine should be adopted which provides for an exercise session on at least five days per week, and preferably (if the opportunity exists) six or even seven days. A routine can readily be devised which hits every major body-part in a thorough way twice per week. Boredom and overtraining can be avoided by devoting one or two exercise days mainly to, say, aerobic training while the other days can concentrate on working, say, one upper and one lower body-part really hard.

Those who have undertaken such a regime usually find, after a month or two, that the body actually begins to crave its daily dose of exercise and that, far from tiring the body, this kind of schedule actually makes them feel more alert both physically and mentally. For the six- or seven-day trainer, an occasional day off can readily be accommodated particularly if it is devoted to other forms of physical activity (e.g. social sport or working in the garden), and may even be found beneficial. Some people find that a two- or three-day break every two weeks is helpful, and that they return to their daily (or near-daily) exercise schedule with renewed vigour and enthusiasm. Longer breaks, such as occur while on holiday, are certainly not excluded though the effect will usually be felt when the trainer returns to the normal schedule and notices a loss of stamina and some muscle soreness; these effects, however, are usually not long-lasting if the break has been only for a week or two. Truly dedicated trainers will usually attempt to do at least some light exercise while on holidays. Some have even been known to take a set of weights with them, although most will usually prefer to improvise using whatever aids come to hand if they are not near a gym.

The training schedule adopted obviously needs to be appropriate to the trainer's age, degree of fitness and stage of training. Above all, it is essential to listen to one's body, noting the types and frequency of exercise to which it responds best and the recuperation periods it requires in order to perform at its optimum capacity. In this sense, the alert and well-informed weight trainer becomes his or her own most attentive and perceptive personal instructor.

14 Training modes

In this chapter we discuss the three chief modes of training with weights, each of which has an important role to play as part of a total training regime. These are generally known as *isotonic, aerobic* and *isometric* training.

Isotonic weight training

This is the most common form of weight training, involving the movement of a weight or other resistant object through a cycle or range of motion exercises using concentric and eccentric muscular contractions. The mechanical and physiological effects of this form of exercise were described in Part I of this book, but a list of isotonic exercises for the various body-parts and muscle-groups is not provided here as you can find a detailed account of the standard exercises in practically all of the available books on weight training. The best overall guide to the performance mechanics of isotonic weight routines is undoubtedly *The Encyclopedia of Modern Bodybuilding* by Arnold Schwarzenegger and Bill Dobbins (London, Pelham Books, 1985). Three works by Robert Kennedy (all published by Sterling Books, New York) will also be found helpful to those seeking to maximise muscle growth: *Hardcore Bodybuilding* (1982), *Beef It!* (1983) and, especially, *Reps!* (1985).

The Matrix exercises described in Part IV of this book make highly specific uses of isotonic (and other) exercise movements as part of the total array of inter-related kinetic forces to which each muscle-group is exposed. In the present section, we deal with some of the general issues connected with isotonic weight training *outside* the Matrix system. These issues may perhaps best be summed up in the three most frequently asked questions in the world of weight training: how many reps? how many sets? how much weight?

The first point that needs to be made is that the three questions are so closely inter-related as to be, in one sense, merely three aspects of a single question: there can be no meaningful answer to any one of them in the absence of answers to the other two. Perhaps the most helpful way of approaching this issue is to consider two extreme cases in the spectrum of weight users. The first is that of the inexperienced trainer, who has suddenly decided to get fit and wanders into the gym having had no instruction in weight training. All experienced gym users have observed this type of trainer who will usually cast a cursory eye on what others are doing, then pick up a couple of weights and start moving them about. More often than not, the weights chosen will be so light that they can have no possible effect in bringing the muscle into a state of full contraction. It can usually be safely predicted that, unless this trainer receives some instruction from an experienced and knowledgeable weight user, he or she will have disappeared from the gym within a week or two, having found the experience (for good reason) to be totally futile.

At the other extreme is the case of the person who has been training with total regularity for a number of years and yet has shown little muscle gain. He (for it is usually a male) may use quite heavy weights and work all body-parts for up to a couple of hours at a stretch, yet never seems to improve, presumably expecting that one day the hoped-for 'breakthrough' will occur. This trainer usually does exactly the same workout, and close examination would reveal that what he does is throw the weights around in 'cheating' movements performed over and over

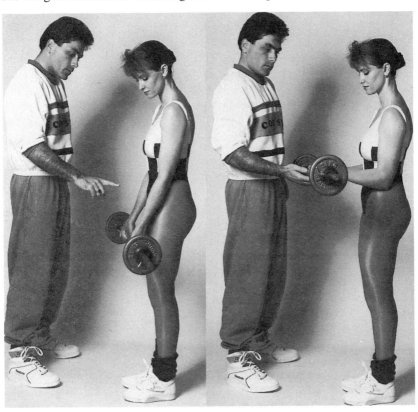

Effective training requires a knowledge of 'correct form'.

again until he tires of one exercise and passes on to the next. None of the movements is performed in the way that will concentrate the overload on the target muscles and maximise the intensity of the contraction, even though quite heavy weights are used.

Between these two extremes there lies a whole continuum of weight use, some of it effective, some of it much less so. How, then, do we identify the correct formula?

The first principle to be observed is that of 'correct form'. The trainer needs to understand the mechanical principles of muscle contraction, so that each movement can be performed in strict style, using only the target muscle-group (i.e. the muscle to be developed and its natural antagonists). Biceps curls and triceps pushdowns, for instance, require that only the forearm should move, the upper arm remaining stationary throughout the movement; deltoid lateral raises require that the weight should be moved by the upper arm, not flung out from the body by the use of the forearm.

Once the mechanics of each movement are understood, a good starting point is to do sets of ten repetitions. The weight chosen should be one which can be comfortably lifted for seven repetitions, so that the last three require an amount of effort which is experienced as a noticeable stress on the muscles, while still allowing the movement to be performed strictly. If this feeling of stress is not experienced in the final reps of the set, the weight should be increased. As the learner gains strength, the weight should be gradually made heavier: it is quite useless to stick with the weights with which the learner first began, and most trainers will find that in a month or so they can increase their weights by at least 25 per cent compared to those with which they started. The increases in weight will gradually taper off, of course, as the trainer approaches the maximum lift of which he or she is capable, but all too many trainers prefer the comfort of a weight they can lift easily to the challenge of a heavier weight which they would be capable of managing if they were prepared to withstand just a little more muscular stress.

Although most beginners will find that three sets done in this way will give them some muscle gain, they should move as soon as possible to a more sophisticated way of calculating the number of sets they will need to perform to maintain their progress. One approach to this calculation is to use the first set as a warm-up set, which stresses the target muscle only on the last three repetitions. The remaining sets should then be organised in such a way that the final set works the target muscle to 'failure' (i.e. you feel that you simply cannot do another rep). In general, the weight used should be such that this failure point is reached by the end of the fourth set; if you can still perform another few reps after this set, you are not using enough weight.

As the trainer advances, the pause between sets should be reduced as far as possible, preferably to between 15 and 30 seconds. The time for rest is between body-parts, not between sets devoted to the same body-part. In this way, the intensity of the workout is maximised, a critical factor in its efficiency. As some experienced trainers point out, 'You can train hard or you can train long, but not both.' It is over-simplistic to assume that if four sets can achieve results, then eight sets must double the results: it is far better to do four sets at maximum intensity, with very short breaks between them and failure at the end of the last set, than to spread out the sets over a longer period of time. The latter method will be far more comfortable, but this is precisely because it reduces the muscular effort and thus the muscle gain.

While the above suggestions provide a general rule-of-thumb, a number of variations are worth considering. Two of these are as follows:

- *Increased reps*   Some muscles (e.g. the calves) respond well to sets consisting of a high number of reps, and certain exercises performed to improve definition (e.g. pec-deck flyes) can also be effective if performed in high-rep mode. If, say, a set of 30 reps is being undertaken, the weight should be such that the first ten are relatively painless, the second ten produce a good pump, and the final ten are distinctly painful. High-rep sets done with too light a weight are practically useless.
- *Increased sets*   We have seen that, if performed with sufficient intensity, only three or four sets per exercise are required. Beyond this, it is better to move to a different exercise for the same body-part rather than add further identical sets. Advanced trainers will sometimes add a third and even fourth exercise for the target body-part, but beginning and intermediate trainers will achieve better results by limiting the number of exercises and increasing their intensity.

A number of other variations in isotonic training will be found in the next chapter.

Aerobic weight training

What is the distinction between aerobic and anaerobic exercise? Researchers have not found it easy to answer this question, for they have traditionally tried to do so by trying to identify two distinct metabolic processes, one of which could be engaged by aerobic exercise, the other by anaerobic exercise. The physiological truth is that there is no exercise that can be defined as wholly aerobic or anaerobic. Instead of thinking of two different concepts, it is more instructive to consider aerobic and anaerobic exercises as simply end-points on the same continuum. While body cells have aerobic and anaerobic energy utilisation pathways, they are not logically dependent on one another.

Aerobic exercise causes the body to utilise more oxygen than anaerobic exercise, but both forms of exercise increase oxygen intake. Aerobic training also tends more effectively, though not exclusively, to utilise body fat as the primary source of energy. Depending on the duration of the exercise, its intensity and the amount of an individual's body fat, aerobic training can also, as can anaerobic, burn glycogen as a source of sustained energy. It is, however, the sustained elevation of body temperature and pulse in respect of oxygen increase which is the key factor associated with aerobic exercise and in this regard it is of course true that certain exercises are more conducive to the production of aerobic effects than others.

Aerobic exercise in the form of dance, for example, assists in the reduction of body fat, though the submaximal nature of the activity does little to enhance muscular development. As a toning exercise, however aerobics is highly efficacious. For quality muscular development, aerobics can thus be effectively combined with weight training. Indeed, it is worth noting that recent research has established that unless the development of strength is concomitant with the acquisition of flexibility, the joints can actually become weakened from the stretching processes entailed by flexibility movements. Development of the muscle areas surrounding the joints assists in diminishing the chance of injury to the joint which can be caused by aerobic running, jumping or stretching movements. In this case, weight training can be used to enhance the effectiveness of aerobics.

The cardio-respiratory benefits of aerobics are well established. The volume of blood pumped by the heart with every beat is increased, which means that the heart has to beat fewer times (i.e. expend less effort) to achieve the same amount of work. The slower a heart beats the longer its owner is likely to live. Recovery time of pulse is also considerably more efficient in those who regularly include aerobics as part of their weight-lifting routine. Moreover, the resting heart rate is substantially lowered by aerobic training, as is blood pressure. Recent research has also shown that libido and sexual performance can be significantly improved and extended by aerobic training. And of course there is for the competitive bodybuilder who includes aerobics as part of his or her training program, the added benefit of a body finely honed and delineated and ready for competition.

There are two major ways in which aerobic exercise can be combined with so-called anaerobic exercise in a total fitness program. One is to devote a number of sessions per week to those forms of non-weight exercise usually described as aerobic either by joining the aerobics groups which have become popular in recent years and include gymnastic or dance movements in their vigorous programs of stretching, bending and on-the-spot running, or through sports which involve fast movement and significant demands on the cardiovascular system (squash, cycling, swimming, etc.), or simply by doing various running exercises from jogging through to sprinting or short and middle-distance running. Some of these activities can be undertaken as one element of a complete session which also involves weight training, while others are best engaged in on separate days from the weight workout.

The second way is to make the aerobic work part of the weight training itself. This method of training is a long-standing practice amongst bodybuilders, and sometimes takes a form known as circuit training. The main principle here is that the exercises performed are the standard weight exercises, but the stress 'is on high repetitions with minimum pauses between sets. Aerobic weight exercises are generally movements which involve major or large muscle groups, such as the legs or chest area. They are movements which can be performed submaximally (i.e. not requiring movement to failure or exhaustion) so as to permit the systematic and sustained elevation of cardio-respiratory functions. This is why aerobic exercise requires that the workloads undertaken by the body are of a sufficiently low intensity to allow their unabated continuation for the appropriate duration.

This is also why variety of movement in an aerobics routine is not simply a matter of warding off boredom. By changing exercises, it becomes possible to regulate the heart rate and blood pressure without overtaxing and fatiguing any one particular muscle area. Unfortunately, many alleged aerobic routines fail to be aerobic in just this way. The emphasis on one or even a few prolonged movements gives rise to what might be called endurance exercises, not aerobic exercises. Prolonged activity on one muscle-group exhausts the muscles by forcing the conversion of glucose molecules into molecules of lactic acid, thus making it difficult to ensure that the pulse does not fluctuate. Insofar as maximal aerobic benefit comes from elevating the heart rate to 75–85 per cent of its pulsive capacity for approximately 20 minutes, the fluctuation of pulse during the 20-minute period can impede the desired result. For this reason, each muscle-group should be worked for only a short time (a minute or so), with light weights and vigorous, though not jerky, movements.

One of the most effective aerobic systems of weight training is the peripheral heart action program, or PHA as it came to be called. The program was originally developed by Bob Gajda who won the 1966 Mr America and 1967 Mr World titles by using the system in conjunction with his conventional training. Then a student of exercise physiology, Gajda was inspired by a lecture on peripheral heart action given by one of his professors. Peripheral heart action refers to a process whereby blood circulates through the arms and legs through a series of muscle contractions which push the blood past one-way valves in the arterial system. Extending the principle, Gajda proposed that numerous muscle contractions across the entire body would further increase blood circulation while minimising overall body fatigue. To stimulate these contractions, a series of 10–12 exercises was deployed with minimum rest between them. Set out below is a PHA routine which can be performed three times per week.

Peripheral Heart Action Program

Monday: Series I
1 Leg press: 1 set of 10–15 reps.
  No rest
2 Incline situps: 1 set of 20–30 reps.
  No rest
3 Bench press: 1 set of 10–12 reps.
  No rest
4 Calf raises: 1 set of 15–20 reps.
  No rest
5 Bent over rows with barbell: 1 set of 12–15 reps.

Having completed the first series, you simply pause for three minutes then repeat the entire series; pause three minutes and repeat, continuing in this way until 5 sets have been completed.

Wednesday: Series II (Note the change of set sequence).
1 Squats: 5 sets of 10–15 reps with a one minute pause between the sets.
  No rest
2 Press behind the neck: 5 sets of 10–12 reps with a one minute pause between the sets.
  No rest
3 Barbell curl: 5 sets of 10–12 reps with a one minute pause between the sets.
  No rest
4 Lying triceps extension: 5 sets of 8–12 reps with a one minute pause between the sets.
  No rest
5 Lat pulldown: 5 sets of 12–15 reps with a one minute pause between the sets.

Friday: Series III (Note the change of set sequence)
1 Incline bench press: 1 set of 15–18 reps.
  No rest
2 Seated leg extension: 1 set of 18–20 reps.
  No rest
3 Dumbbell side laterals: 1 set of 12–15 reps.
  No rest
4 Bent arm pullover: 1 set of 12–15 reps.
  No rest
5 Standing alternating dumbbell curls: 1 set of 12–15 reps.

As with the first and second series, having completed the third series, you simply pause for three minutes then repeat the entire series; pause three minutes and repeat again, continuing in this way until you have completed 5 sets of each of the exercises in the series.

In more advanced PHA training, all the different exercises are performed on the same day during a single training session. Although the PHA system works well to improve cardiovascular fitness as a result of its aerobic circuit basis, one disadvantage of the routine is the length of time taken to complete the day's training. In addition to the more sophisticated techniques incorporated in Matrix training, the brief period of actual exercise time required by the Matrix Principle provides a decided efficiency advantage over conventional programs including the PHA. While maximising muscular development and strength gains, Matrix training minimises both the daily training time required and the overall period during which gains are made.

Isometric weight training

Isotonic exercise, as we saw above, involves lifting, pushing or pulling a weight through a cycle or range of motion exercises by means of muscular contraction. As such, it is usually distinguished from isometric (or resistive) exercise, in which the muscles are contracted but there is no movement of the limb or limbs involved. In the first case, it is supposed (not entirely accurately) that the muscle retains the *same tone* or intensity of contraction throughout the range of movement of the limb, whereas in an isometric contraction the muscle retains the *same length* (in Greek, *isos metros*) since the limb does not move.

Isometric exercise was popularised in the early 1950s by the German scientists Hettinger and Moller, and was soon being promoted in training literature as a simple means of exercising without the need for weights. The busy executive was urged to take time out in the office to contract various muscle-groups, using perhaps a desk or the wall for resistance, and to concentrate on the muscle-group being used, forcing the blood-flow into these particular muscles as hard as possible.

The promoters of isometric exercise claimed (with a degree of justification) to have observed that a large number of men (e.g. road workers) who were involved daily in hard physical labour requiring vigorous movement of the limbs often showed surprisingly little muscular development. Similarly, laboratory experiments in which a frog was strapped to a board, with one leg immobile in splints and the other free to flex and move, had led to a finding opposite to that which the researchers expected: it was the immobile leg, rather than the one which was being actively exercised, that developed the larger muscles.

The conclusion was drawn that the very fact of straining a muscle against an immovable object led to an increase in size and strength equal to or greater than what would have been achieved by engagement in strenuous exercise involving movement. It was postulated that when a muscle strained against an immovable object for even a short period, it enjoyed a suffusion of blood which flushed and nourished the cells.

Various exercises were therefore devised which would pit human muscles against an immovable object, and programs were set up

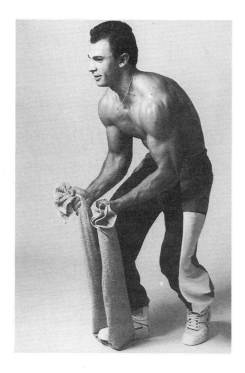

Isometric training—using, for example, a towel to provide resistance—can be a helpful adjunct to other exercise modes.

involving the use of minimal equipment (a towel or a length of rope) or no equipment at all. Physical instructors in the US armed forces were soon using the new isometric methods in their training programs, and the attraction of being able to exercise at home, in the office or even in bed made isometrics a popular fad for some years. Exaggerated claims were made for the method, which some saw as replacing weight training for physical fitness and muscular development. In time, the fashion passed, and there were even attempts at debunking it, for instance by the claim that it was a myth that had been spread to the USA by Soviet athletic trainers as being the reason for the greater size and strength of their athletes, in order to mask the 'real' secret of their success, namely the use of anabolic steroids which were being introduced about that time.

With the benefit of hindsight, it is now possible to give a more accurate and balanced assessment of the effectiveness of isometric exercise. Whilst exaggerated claims of outstanding fitness or development resulting from a few minutes a day in the home or office have rightly been discredited, nonetheless the basic principle (the concentrated flexing of a muscle whilst it is held motionless against a counter-balancing force) has been generally accepted as a useful means of stimulating development. In addition to the physiological factor of suffusion mentioned above (a factor which can also brought into play in other forms of exercise), isometric contraction—flexing or tensing—is today seen as a useful adjunct to, if by no means a replacement for, the more traditional isotonic exercise involved in weight training.

There are two main methods of performing isometric exercise:

- by exertion against an immovable object or load—type (a) e.g. pushing up against a door frame or exertion against a fixed bar on the power rack;
- by contractions of both agonist and antagonist muscles, a method sometimes referred to as dynamic tension—type (b) e.g. pushing the hands together, contracting the biceps with hands clasped and one arm working against the resistance of the other.

A third form of isometric tension is that used by competitive bodybuilders in their performance of the compulsory poses and the stationary poses included in 'free posing'. Performing and practising these poses is also a means used by bodybuilders for improving muscle definition. This is generally a form of non-resistive isometric tension, relying purely on the voluntary flexing of muscles, though in certain poses (e.g. side chest, side triceps) a form of dynamic tension is also used.

Simple isometric exercises of types (a) and (b) include:

- clasping a book between the palms of both hands and pressing inwards (for the pectoral muscles);
- placing the hands under a table-top, with elbows bent, and pushing the palms upwards (for the biceps);
- in a seated position, placing the knees under a desk-top and pushing upwards on the balls of the feet (for the calves);
- in a seated position, placing the hands under the chair and pulling upwards with both hands (for the triceps);
- holding in both hands a towel looped under one foot, and pulling upwards (for the biceps)

The list of possible exercises performed in this way is almost endless, depending solely on the imagination of the exerciser and the availability of a towel, chair, piece of rope, or doorway. Various exercise devices, such as Bullworkers, 'power-crushers' and specially designed isometric T-bars are also suitable for this type of resistance work.

The chief benefit of isometric exercise is that it enables a muscle to be fully contracted at highly specific angles, whereas in isotonic movements the leverage factor means that a weight which may fully contract the target muscle at one point of the movement may not contract it fully at other points. As muscles are stronger in a position of stasis than in concentric contraction (i.e. they can 'hold' more weight at any one point in the muscle's range of motion than they can positively lift to that point), the isometric tension is able to produce a greater contraction at that specific point than could be achieved in the course of a concentric movement.

By the same token, however, because the isometric tension is specific to one particular point in the total range of muscle movement involved in any given exercise, it is imperative for overall development to per-

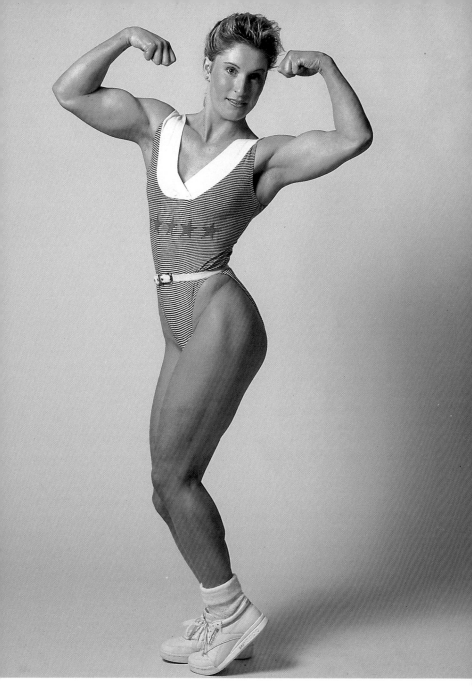

Shown on the following pages are a number of exercisers of various ages who include Matrix training as part of their regular weight workouts. Although their goals are very different, ranging from general fitness to success in competitive bodybuilding, each of them has benefited from the Matrix routines explained in the final section of this book.

Melissa Croft has won several national titles in women's bodybuilding. She demonstrates how muscular development and femininity can be complementary rather than opposite qualities.

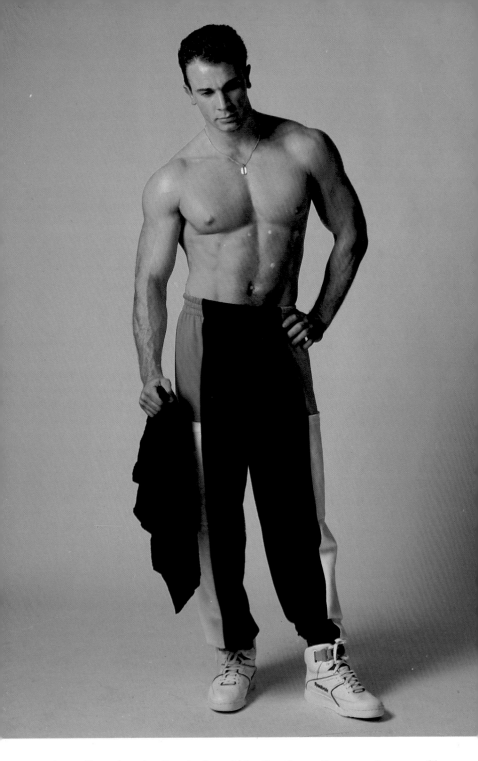

Lauro Sottovia trains 'for the fun of it' rather than with an eye to competition.
Relatively short training sessions of high intensity keep him in superb shape as well
as maintaining the cardiovascular fitness he needs as a keen soccer player.

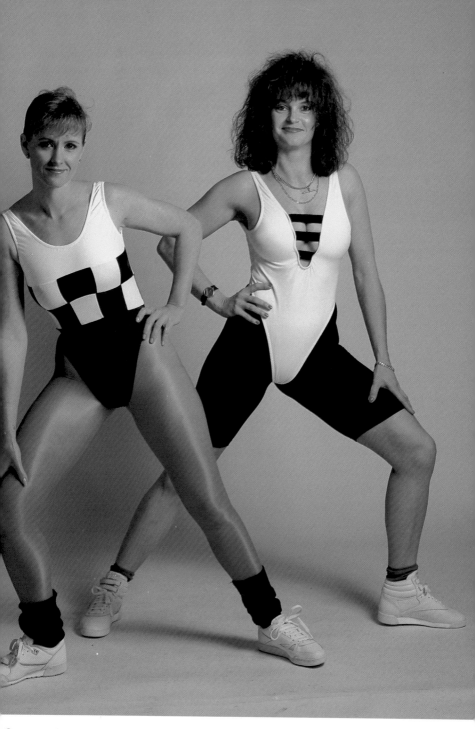

Suzanne Kondraki and Kim Emsermann have found that a combination of aerobic exercise and Matrix weight training keeps their figures trim and attractive by maintaining muscle-tone and lowering body-fat levels without recourse to excessive dieting.

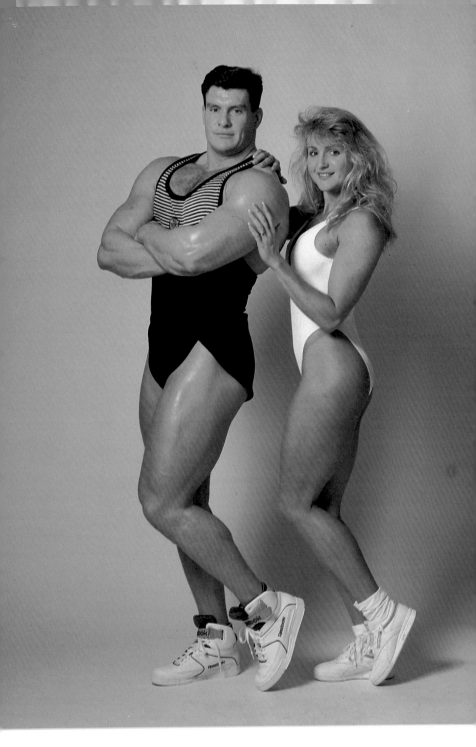

Paul and Monica Haslam are a husband-and-wife team who run a commercial gymnasium. The need to be seen as credible role-models by their pupils requires them to remain in peak physical condition the year round.

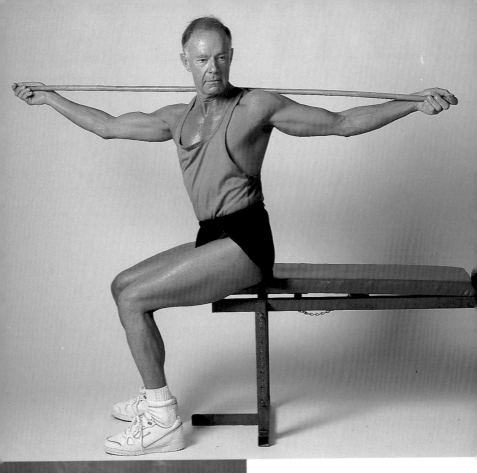

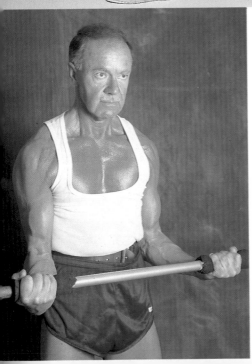

Ken Dutton is a senior academic and administrator in his fifties, who takes time out to train six days a week. He believes that the time spent on exercise is more than repaid by the increased mental efficiency and enhanced concentration that result.

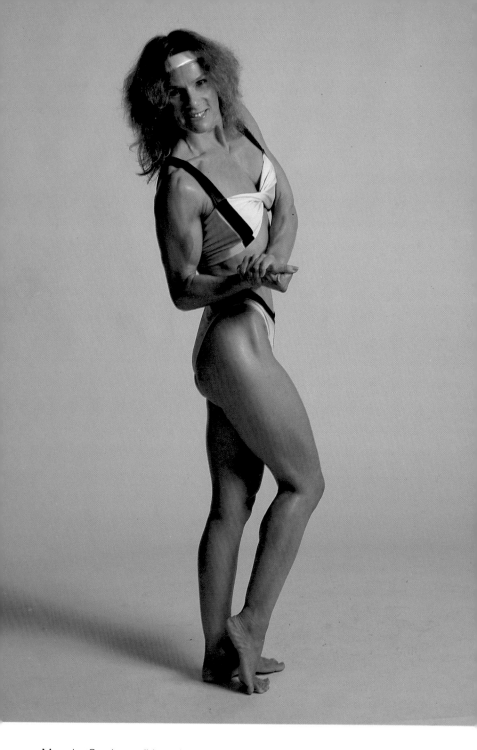

Marysha Stephens did not begin weight training till her thirties. In addition to running a business with her husband and bringing up a family, she has managed to win numerous bodybuilding and powerlifting competitions owing to the concentrated efficiency of Matrix training.

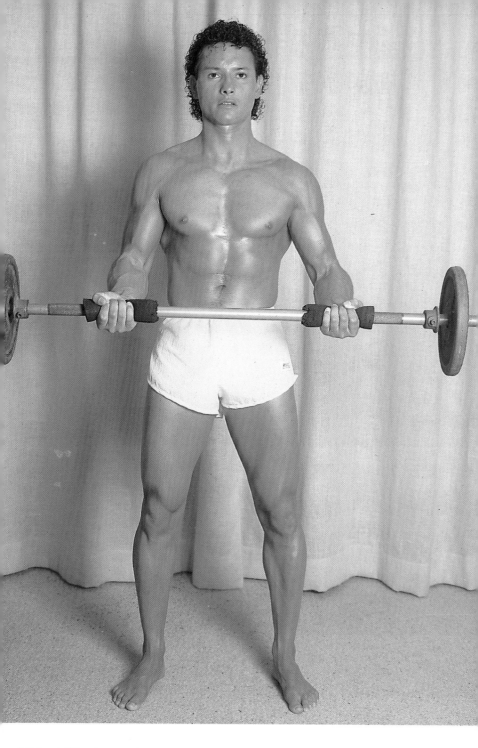

Michael Gillies is a professional entertainer whose job requires him to keep in good shape. When his performance schedule precludes regular gym workouts, he uses Matrix training at home with simple weights, supplemented by a more extensive workout in the gym when opportunity allows.

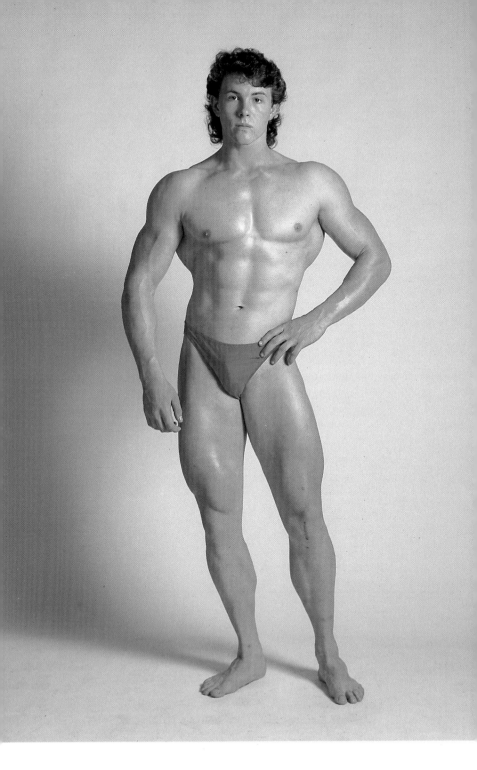

Jamie Roberts is starting out on a competitive bodybuilding career and has already won a number of Australian regional titles in the junior division. A natural mesomorph, he has a bright future in competition.

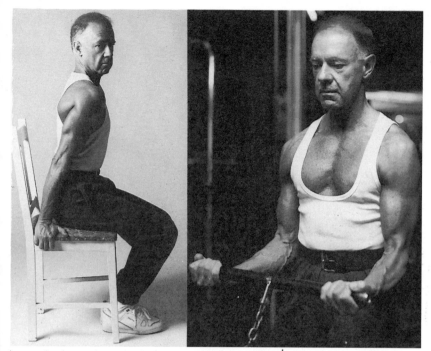

Isometric contractions can be performed using a chair or an isometric T-bar, and are a particularly effective training method for older exercisers.

form each isometric exercise in a variety of positions. Experimentation in isometric training has indicated that a minimum of three and a maximum of twelve positions provide the best results. Each exercise should consist of at least three positons: near the start of the movement, half-way into the movement, and near the end of the movement. Each position is held at maximum tension for between six and twelve seconds.

Three particularly good isometric exercises for the development of strength are the squat, bench press and bent-legged deadlift. Below is an example of the way in which to perform isometric squats. The principles of performance indicated can simply be extended to the bench press and the bent-legged deadlift.

A power rack is ideally suited to the performance of isometric resistance training. Set the bar to a position about 15 cm (6 in) below the shoulder level. By wrapping a towel around the bar, you can reduce the pressure it will place on the trapezius muscles which protect the back of the neck. Inhale deeply prior to taking a position under the bar and, when set, hold your breath for a 2–3 second period while building up tension against the bar. Your full exertion against the bar of 6–12 seconds should be accompanied by a slow exhalation of breath using abdominal contraction. Finish the isometric by reducing the exertion over a 2–3 second period, then inhale normally. This completes one

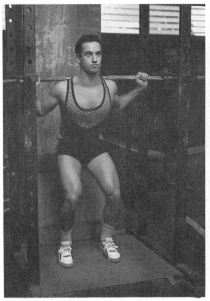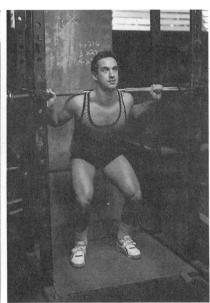

Isometric squats using the power rack.

repetition, and depending upon your condition, you should perform between 5 and 10 repetitions with 30–60 seconds between the repetitions. For the second set of isometric squats the fixed bar is lowered another 15 cm (6 in), give or take variations of support spacing on the power rack, and the same exertion or static pressing in the squat position is repeated as above. The bar is lowered systematically by 15 cm (6 in) for the third and remaining sets until it is adjusted in the power rack at the full squat position. If you are interested in a real challenge, you can work your way back to the upright starting position using the same system. As indicated earlier, the bench press and deadlift isometrics can be performed similarly on the power rack.

The slow build-up to full exertion and subsequent period of relaxation is required to minimise injury and reflects the physiological state of variable muscle tension which exists in the body during actual training. Muscle fatigue accelerates at a rate proportional to the duration of the exertion, and the concentration required to maintain intensity also deteriorates during extended exertions, particularly with the onset of muscle fatigue. Experience indicates that periods of 6–12 seconds maximum exertion yield substantial results and minimise both general body fatigue and mental fatigue. The timing and intensity of isometric training can be correlated with the anaerobic phosphate energy system of the body which supplies a high power output during the first 10–12 seconds of activity.

15 Training techniques

Having given a general outline of the chief modes of weight training, we can go on to discuss a number of specific techniques which enable the standard isotonic workout to be varied so as to maximise its effectiveness in building muscle.

A few remarks should be made by way of introduction. We have seen that the amount of weight required in weight training varies considerably, depending on the body-part being exercised, the age, weight, sex, somatotype and stage of training of the person exercising, and the type of exercise being performed (heavy weights being unsuitable, for example, for aerobic training). The traditional approach has been to divide weight training into two basic kinds: high-weight low-rep, and low-weight high-rep training. We have already referred to some of the misconceptions underlying this simplistic distinction, particularly the view that only one of these is suitable for maximum muscle growth. The point to note here is that both types of training have their place, and that certain heavy-weight exercises, in particular squats, bench press, calf raises and to a certain extent biceps and triceps exercises, can be highly effective muscle builders if carried out correctly.

The importance of correct technique is crucial if muscle strain and ligament injury are to be avoided. Only those with a knowledge of powerlifting techniques are advised to attempt heavy squats and heavy bench presses, for instance, as incorrect placement or angle of lift can (and all too often does) cause spinal injuries and, in the case of squats, knee and hip injuries. Trainers who have the requisite strength and knowledge of technique will find it useful to test their level of strength on such exercises, and to compete against one another or against themselves in matching or exceeding their previous maximum weight for these lifts. The massive chest and upper-leg development acquired by competitive powerlifters indicates the effectiveness of these exercises as muscle builders.

Heavy weights are not, however, the key to effective weight training. The crucial factor lies in the *maximum stimulation of the muscles* by

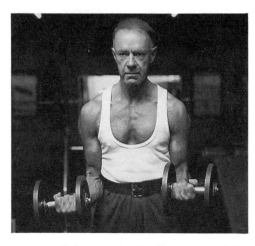

Slow-repetition training can make even light weights a powerful means of providing resistance to the muscles.

means of the overload effect: a combination of sufficient weight resistance and repeated contraction. This combination brings about an accumulation of fatigue products which so overload the muscle system's feed-in and drain-off lines that the system undergoes an adaptive response by expanding in size in order to cope with future stresses of a similar kind. This expansion, as we have seen, takes place during periods of recuperation.

We noted earlier that this expansion of the muscle system is better promoted by repeated muscle contraction, preferably of a number of sets each building upon the last, than by a small number of repetitions, even at maximum intensity. More than one set is required in order to tax fully the incoming and outgoing blood vessels which supply new fuel and remove the waste accumulation. Low repetitions, even at maximum resistance, do not encourage the widening of vascular channels (or increase in muscle size) as effectively as does the intense stimulation caused by repeated contraction against a moderate resistance which builds up to a point of complete overload.

In this chapter we suggest a number of training techniques which can be used to foster and intensify the overload effect. Some of them are more suitable for advanced trainers, others for those who for one reason or another are unable to undertake high-intensity work with moderate weights. All of them, however, can be used effectively as variations on the standard isotonic routine described earlier. The techniques they employ include some which are incorporated into the Matrix workouts (found in Part IV), which combine them with other techniques in specific sequences and rotating sets to increase their intensity and effectiveness to a degree which cannot be matched by standard training methods.

Slow repetitions

It is a basic tenet of weight training that the weight should be raised and lowered in a relatively slow and deliberate fashion, without jerking or throwing it about. It has been shown in numerous experiments that once the speed of the weight's movement exceeds a certain rate, the force of momentum takes over and the muscular contraction is consequently diminished. Avoiding momentum enables the trainer to gain the maximum degree of muscle stimulation for the movement of a given weight by ensuring that all muscle fibres are thoroughly engaged instead of understressing some and overstressing others. It also reduces the risk of tendon injury which can be caused by the uncontrolled movement of too heavy a weight.

One method of increasing the effectiveness of deliberate and controlled weight movement without increasing the weight is simply to increase the time taken to perform the movements themselves. An important underlying principle of this slow-repetition training is that, just as we can hold in a stationary position a heavier weight than we can lift to that position, so we can move in a negative (or eccentric) movement a heavier weight than we can either hold stationary or raise in a positive (or concentric) contraction. For this reason, it is sometimes recommended that the lowering of a weight should take a little longer than the raising of the weight. In slow-repetition training, however, the opposite holds true. For any given weight, the additional resistance required to perform the positive (or weaker) movement slowly will not be called upon in the negative (or stronger) movement: since the muscle is stronger in the negative phase, the weight will simply not be heavy enough, and too slow a negative movement will thus allow the muscle to rest slightly. For this reason, the negative movement should be performed less slowly than the positive, in order to oblige the muscle to maintain the intensity of its contraction rather than relaxing on the stronger phase of the exercise.

The first step in slow-repetition training is to count the time you are presently taking to perform these movements. (The simplest method of counting seconds is to count to yourself 'One thousand and one, one thousand and two' etc.) Most trainers will probably be surprised to observe that they are taking as little as one second on each of the raising and lowering movements.

The next step is to increase deliberately the time your are taking, especially on the positive movement. Three seconds up, and one or two seconds down, will be the initial goal, and if you can reach it easily you should try four seconds up and two seconds down. For most trainers, a set performed in this way with the weights they normally use will prove extremely painful or even impossible; if this is the case, you should select a weight light enough to enable you to perform three or four sets while strictly maintaining the time-count.

Using the same (lighter) weights, you can then move on in subsequent workouts to sets involving six seconds up, two or three seconds down; eight seconds up, three seconds down; and so on. A ten-second positive and four-second negative movement will generally be found to be the maximum that can usefully be performed. Biceps curls, triceps push-downs, lat pulldowns, leg extensions and leg curls lend themselves especially well to slow-repetition training, but it can be extended to a variety of other standard weight exercises.

The slow-repetition technique will be found to produce a surprising degree of muscle pump even with quite light weights, and will also accustom the trainer to slowing down the reps even in standard exercises. As with other forms of isotonic training, the pauses between sets should be as brief as possible, and it may be helpful to have a set of lighter weights standing by in case the weights used for the first two sets feel too heavy to move at the same slow speed in the third and fourth sets. As always, the aim should be to reach a point of failure at the end of the final set.

Part repetitions

A well-known training method is the '21' system. For barbell curls, for example, this method involves doing seven reps in which the barbell is lifted only half-way up from the starting position to the top of the movement, then lowered again; this is followed immediately by seven reps in which the barbell is lifted from the half-way point to the top of the movement; and again followed immediately by seven full reps. This makes a total set of 21 repetitions.

Many different weight exercises (e.g. triceps pushdowns, lat pull-downs, leg presses, leg extensions etc.) can be performed in this way, and the muscle pump is intense. The effect of this exercise is produced by the fact that a higher number of reps is possible than if the same 'full' movement was used throughout. Each of the two parts of the movement works the target muscle in a slightly different way, pre-stressing it so that it responds more intensely to the full pump in the final seven reps. So concentrated is this exercise that, if performed with sufficient weight, failure will be achieved by the end of the second set.

Not only are the part-reps used in the '21' method incorporated in a more sophisticated way in Matrix training, they were historically a forerunner of the Matrix system itself. When, as a childhood body-builder, R. S. Laura found himself unable to complete full sets of 10 curls with the weight he was using, he turned to using a lighter weight and performing upper and lower half-curls followed by full curls, with equal or better results. The sets of seven were chosen because that was his age at the time, the total of 21 representing his ambition (later realised) to be a world champion weightlifter by that age. After some initial scepticism, his elder brother James Laura adopted this training method and later introduced it into a number of health studios which he managed in California, where it was soon taken up by a number of Californian bodybuilders and has since become a standard technique.

The '21' system takes advantage of the physiological fact that, as the limbs are moved, the muscles controlling them are subjected to a continuum of different stresses. At each point in the movement, the

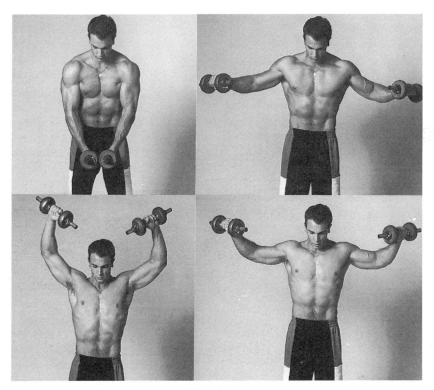

The '21' method involves performing one half of a movement (*top pair*), then the other half (*lower pair*) before performing the complete movement. There are 7 repetitions in each of the three phases of the set, making a total of 21 repetitions.

muscle configuration or bunching pattern is slightly different, and this is why we observed in relation to isometric exercise that a number of different tension positions were needed for each exercise. The bunching pattern of the biceps near the start of the curl, for instance, is entirely different from that which it adopts at the top of the movement. In the '21' system, the effort is concentrated intensively, first on one section of contracted muscle, then on another, thus eliminating the relaxation effect which takes place when other muscle fibres take over the load.

The same holds true for muscle-groups as for individual muscles. If you observe from behind an advanced bodybuilder doing lat pulldowns, particularly if they are done slowly, you will notice how the muscular configuration of the upper back changes during the performance of the movement. The various muscles involved—teres major, rhomboids and infraspinatus, and trapezius—all change their particular bunching patterns as first one, then another, comes more into play to take the load. It is for this reason that some bodybuilders occasionally like to try a variation on the '21' system whereby they work only one short range of the movement at a time, pulling the bar through as little as 30 cm (12 in) or so of its total range of movement for each set of repetitions before finishing off with a set of full repetitions. Like the standard '21' exercises, this concentrates muscle fibre stimulation in a highly specific way.

Ladders

Sometimes known by different names (pyramids, step bombing), this is a training technique which can be adapted to a variety of forms. Basically, it involves increasing or decreasing the weight during the course of what amounts to a very long continuous set (sometimes known as a giant set), and for that reason is best undertaken with the assistance of a training partner so as to minimise the delay and loss of pump while the trainer changes the weights. In those ladder exercises where the weight is progressively increased, the reps are necessarily decreased; similarly, in those where the weight is progressively decreased, the number of reps is deliberately increased.

In its simplest form, the trainer begins with a weight that is light enough to enable a set of ten reps to be performed comfortably. At the end of the set (and within ten seconds of completing it), 5 kg (or 10 lb) are added to the bar and the trainer does a further set; ten reps may again be possible, or the trainer may be able to do only eight or nine. A further 5 kg are added for the next set (again, no more than ten seconds intervening), and the trainer may be able to do no more than four or five reps. The process is continued until only a single rep is possible before failure occurs.

The exercise can also be performed in reverse, either separately from the above exercise or shortly (say, 30 seconds) after it. This time, 5 kg (or 10 lb) are removed with each set until the trainer returns to the original weight, each time doing as many reps as possible. Most barbell exercises (e.g. curls, bench press, overhead press) can be performed using this technique.

A further variation on the ladder principle can be performed with exercises for which a variety of different limb positions is possible. Here, the exercise involves a way of hitting the muscles from different angles which resembles the 'full-range' approach of the Matrix method described in Part IV.

One of the best examples of this is the bench press (done either with free weights or on a machine). The trainer selects a relatively easy weight, and performs five full repetitions with a medium grip (approximately shoulder-width). After a pause of no more than ten seconds, the trainer repeats the same five reps followed immediately by five further reps with a wide grip. For the third set (again after a very short pause), the trainer does five medium-grip, five wide-grip and another five medium-grip reps, all without pause as part of a single set. By this time it may be necessary to lower the weight slightly, either between sets or, if necessary but with great speed, during a set. The fourth set consists of five medium-grip, five wide-grip, five medium-grip and five narrow-grip presses. For the last set, the weight will have to be considerably reduced.

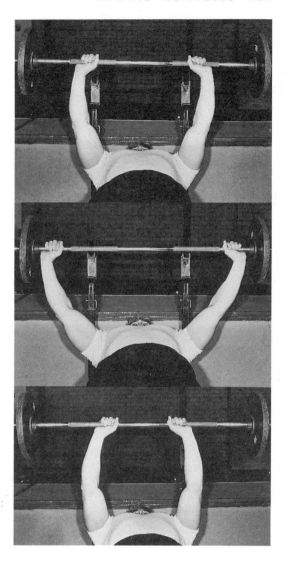

The three grips used in the 'ladder' method bench press: (*top*) medium grip; (*middle*) wide grip; (*bottom*) narrow grip.

This set consists of five medium-grip, five wide-grip, five medium-grip, five narrow-grip and five medium-grip presses. Even advanced trainers will find that, by the end of this final set, they have had to reduce the load to a very light weight indeed (perhaps as little as one or two plates on the bench-press machine), but the resulting pump is little short of phenomenal.

With a combination of common-sense and ingenuity, the ladder principle can be applied to a number of standard weight-training exercises, both for the sake of variety and muscle-shock, and also to provide a method of working the muscle system with extreme intensity and efficiency.

Imaging

We saw in Part I of this book that the important factor in muscle contraction is the degree of resistance encountered by the muscle, and that the message indicating the resistance required is conveyed to the muscle fibres by the neuro-motor system. Obviously, there comes a point at which the weight involved is so heavy that the muscles are unable to respond to the brain's message no matter how hard we try; similarly, tiredness in the muscles may have the same effect even with lighter weights if the number of repetitions is high. Short of 'muscle failure', however, it remains true that the brain can to some extent determine the amount of resistance required of the muscles, irrespective of the actual weight being lifted.

On the basis of this principle, it is possible to simulate the effect of lifting a heavier weight than we are actually lifting. The muscles do not themselves 'know' the heaviness of the weight being used: they know only the message being conveyed to them by the motor nerves. We can take advantage of this principle by using in our training the process known as imaging, in which we deliberately simulate the effect of a weight heavier than the one we are using, or even exercise without weights while simulating the resistance imposed by weight use. The basic technique involved is to set up a mental image of the heavier weight—in simple terms, to 'imagine' it—and perform the exercise as though we were in fact pumping a heavier weight, magnifying the resistance we impose on the exercising muscle. While this may sound a complex approach, it is actually very simple in practice, and the muscle pump it provides can match or even surpass that which is created by the use of heavier weights.

This imaging technique should be distinguished from two other men-

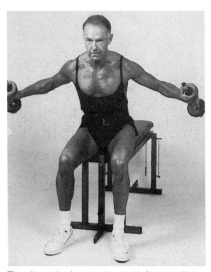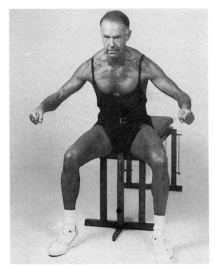

The 'imaging' technique: (*left*) with light weights; (*right*) without weights.

tal control methods which are also a legitimate part of the armoury of weight training. These are, first, the technique of visualising the target muscle as growing larger and larger (a mental suggestion technique successfully used by Arnold Schwarzenegger amongst others), and, second, the form of self-hypnosis used by some bodybuilders and numerous weightlifters whereby they 'will themselves' to lift increasingly heavier weights. The imaging technique described here is not a form of hypnosis or auto-suggestion, so much as a means of exploiting to the full the capacity of muscles to respond to brain signals independently of the actual load placed on them.

The process of using light weights in an imaging technique relies for its effectiveness on our knowing the movement involved and doing it extremely strictly. Let us take, for example, the case of standing (or seated) lateral dumbbell flyes for the middle head of the deltoid. The critical moving part here is the upper arm, which is raised sideways from the shoulder. The trainer should concentrate on the means by which this raising takes place (i.e. the deltoid contraction). The mind should therefore be fixed on the middle head of the deltoid: we need to feel, as far as possible, its squeezing or contraction. The point of doing the movement strictly is to imprint its form in the 'muscle memory', so that when we do it with heavier weights we shall find it easier to avoid cheating.

To develop the mental feel of the movement (i.e. to strengthen the particular neuro-muscular signals involved), the trainer can do a few repetitions with very light weights or even without weights. What goes through the trainer's mind, at each repetition, should not be 'I am raising and lowering my upper arm' but 'I am contracting, then releasing, the middle head of the deltoid'. This mental process is crucial to the success of the imaging technique, and with practice one can gain not only a heightened sense of the target muscle (improved biofeedback), but an increased degree of control over it.

Having acquired the technique, we can create variations to work other muscles in the same general area. For instance, knowing that the upper part of the trapezius contracts during lateral flyes in order to assist the deltoid, we can now do an additional number of sets against the background of a mental 'fix' which tells us: 'I am contracting and releasing the trapezius so as to raise and lower the arms.'

A typical workout in imaging mode might begin with ten reps using moderate weights, to get the feel of the muscle movement. The next few sets will be done with light weights (or even, if need be, without weights) but in each set we will imagine an increasingly heavy weight held in our hands. Sets of 12 or 15 reps will probably be found most useful, and by the seventh or eighth rep in each set we should feel a strong muscle pump. The sets should be continued until muscle tiredness forces us to stop. Amazingly, even without weight, the effect will be felt after a few sets. After a couple of minutes' recuperation, it is helpful to return to the weight we would normally use, and perform two or three standard isotonic sets attempting, as far as possible, to retrieve from the 'muscle memory' the strict movements we were doing earlier. The reason for reverting to 'normal' weights at the end is that muscle pumping (through the imaging technique) does not provide the same degree of overload as that produced by standard weight training: it acts through repeated and increasing stress at submaximal levels rather than through the maximum contractions typical of weight use. By adding a couple of sets of standard weight movements to the imaging movements the full range of stimulation can be applied to the muscles.

Imaging techniques can be devised for a large number of muscle groups, and exercises which work well in this mode include bench flyes, squats, biceps curls and leg extensions. Almost any standard exercise can be adapted to the imaging technique, which is not only effective in its own right but can also assist in the performance of standard weight-training exercises. Though not a substitute for conventional weight training, which alone can provide the degree of overload required for maximum muscle growth, it can be a helpful variant for a short period between bouts of 'regular' weight training, to imprint a strict technique on the muscle memory. It can also assist in promoting definition and provide a means of returning gradually to heavy weight work after suffering a muscle strain or tear. It is particularly useful for those who because of age or physical condition cannot incorporate very intense weight training or a weekly Matrix workout into their exercise regime.

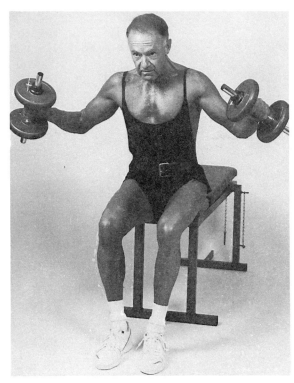

After several sets in 'imaging' mode, the trainer reverts to normal weights.

16 The Matrix Principle at work

Throughout the earlier sections of this book, we have already made passing reference to some of the main features of Matrix training, in so far as they were related to the issues being discussed in individual chapters. In Part I, for instance, we considered some of the mechanical and physiological aspects of muscle contraction which Matrix training seeks to exploit in particular ways. In Part II, we indicated its place as part of a holistic regime of physical fitness and muscle development. In Part III, we have looked at some of the techniques used in conventional training modes which Matrix training takes up and integrates into a total system. It is not our purpose in this chapter to recapitulate the above material but rather to set out what we believe distinguishes the Matrix system from traditional exercise modes.

Recent developments in electron microscopy, combined with a more complete understanding of muscle physiology, have provided insights into the nature of muscle growth which were previously unknown or purely matters of conjecture. The Matrix Principle has been developed in the light of the most recent advances in the field of exercise physiology and refined over more than a decade by a clinical practice of trial and error to achieve an appropriate degree of match between theory and practice.

It is now well established, for example, that muscle cells consist of a number of different components which work in collaboration to bring about body movement and initiate a variety of body functions. Considerable attention has focused upon fast- and slow-twitch fibres as the contractile fibres largely responsible for the growth of skeletal muscle. The basic idea is that different types of training are required in order to stimulate each of the respective fibre-types. The distinction has understandably fuelled the debate on the relative merits of light-weight high-repetition training versus low-repetition heavy-weight training. Training with heavy weights in high-speed movements is believed to stimulate the white fast-twitch fibres, while high-repetition work is supposed to enhance the development of red or slow-twitch fibres. The physiological principle which is presumed to explain this difference of effect is the principle of specific adaptation to imposed demands, otherwise known as the SAID principle, the idea being that you cannot work both fast- and slow-twitch fibres equally effectively with the same type of exercise. Whilst there is an element of truth in this conclusion, it is a truth which has been only partly understood.

From the fact that an exercise is specific, it does not follow that a specific exercise cannot be comprehensive in the stress pattern it places upon a muscle cell. The concept behind the Matrix Principle is that a comprehensive growth response can be achieved by combining a range of specific movements designed to tax the muscle from different angles and in varying modes within a systematic framework of progressive resistance. The result is what we shall describe as deep muscle fibre activation, or the capacity to engage several planes of muscle fibre simultaneously. The pattern of adjustment response imposed upon the muscle is thus 'interplanal', and constantly changing to encourage the muscle to growth.

The reasons it is believed that the Matrix Principle achieves a comprehensive growth response rather than the more limited point-specific response associated with conventional training programs may be summarised as follows:

- Each of the conventional exercises is adapted by introducing partial movements to stress the muscle at the points of axis at which the leverage advantage of the muscle is minimised. This forces the muscle to adapt through gains in size and strength by isolating the points of greatest vulnerability and weakness within the arc of movement. Simply by stopping the barbell at the point of greatest disadvantage and weakness, we have evoked the most significant stress demands which could be placed on the muscle.
- By incorporating into a single exercise several different movements which themselves change from one rep to another, the muscle remains 'confused', in that it is unable to anticipate through its adaptive neural mechanisms the requisite response to the incoming stress. In this regard, Matrix training presupposes the 'muscle confusion' principle.
- By using light weights Matrix training minimises the risk of injury to connective tissues such as ligaments and tendons which are often damaged by training with heavy weights. Similarly, Matrix training reduces the risk of injury to joints and tears to muscles. This makes the system of benefit to exercisers of all ages.
- The precise timing and sequences of sets are designed to challenge the metabolic equilibrium responsible for both weight gain and weight loss. Matrix training can thus be used either to gain weight or to reduce obesity. Another important benefit of the system is that the rapid succession of sets and high reps promotes cardiovascular fitness.
- Although the mechanisms by which muscular growth is actually

stimulated are not altogether clear, it has been demonstrated that muscle-groups which are predominantly interactive are best stimulated to growth by general or group-interactive movements, followed by isolation movements. Matrix training combines general and isolation movements to *pre-exhaust* the support muscles which work in synergy with specific muscles, thus making it easier to isolate specific muscles.

- Matrix training combines into a coherent single exercise sequence a number of the most advanced training principles and techniques. Isotonic, isometric and isokinetic (continuous tension) movements are drawn together into a matrix in which the timing between each repetition and each set is carefully orchestrated to maximise the adaptive response of the mechanisms responsible for accelerated muscle growth.

- By incorporating high-speed and high-intensity movements into a pattern which exhausts the glycogen stores of muscle repeatedly, it is possible that Matrix training encourages hyperplasia or cell-splitting as a prelude to hypertrophy. Whether hyperplasia is the explanation of the success of Matrix training in promoting rapid growth remains a moot point, and it is important to stress that the Matrix Principle does not depend on the validity of hyperplasia as a physiological theory. All that is being claimed here is that the results it exhibits are those which one would expect to find if the theory were valid. The confirmed anabolic effect of Matrix training is not dependent on the cell-splitting theory: it stands on its own as an experimental finding.

Although we have advanced in this chapter some of the theoretical underpinnings of the Matrix Principle, it has not been our purpose in this book to present a new *theory* of weight training so much as a *system*

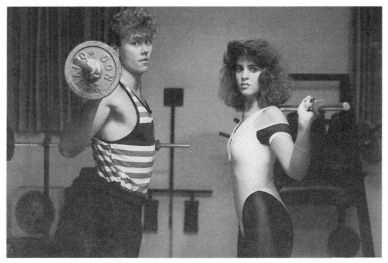

The Matrix Principle does not involve heavy weights: light weights or an unweighted bar can be used, depending on the exerciser's strength.

which has proved itself by its results. We have reproduced just a few of the many testimonials we hold indicating the dramatic results typically experienced by trainers in the clinic where the Matrix Principle has been developed and tested. They strengthen our belief that, like any training method, the Matrix system must ultimately be evaluated on the basis of its outcome in actual practice. The experience of these trainers amongst numerous others may serve to indicate that our claim for the superior effectiveness of the Matrix system over conventional methods has met the most important criterion of all: proven results.

Testimonials

After years of hard work with conventional weight routines, I achieved a level of muscle development that allowed me to place successfully in amateur bodybuilding contests. But it was Matrix training that brought the breakthrough. It gave me the extra size and cuts that I needed to have the edge in professional competition at national and international levels, and I went on to take out the Australasian professional bodybuilding championship. I make regular use of the Matrix Principle in my work as weight-training conditioner for a first-grade Rugby team, and the results have confirmed my own experience of its superiority over other training methods.

Ian Riley
Sydney, NSW

Before I tried the Matrix system I spent several years of hard labour to gain a few kilos of muscle. Within six months of Matrix training I gained more muscle and gains in strength than I did during the previous five years. 'Matrix magic' are the only words for it.

Peter Emsermann
Carey Bay, NSW

I took up weight training in my mid-thirties. It was a sheer stroke of luck that I met Professor Laura, who not only encouraged me to try the Matrix Principle, but to compete using it. Having been introduced to the Matrix system, I have never looked back or felt and looked better. Within the last few years I have won nearly thirty trophies in women's bodybuilding and powerlifting. Anyone looking for rapid progress should be looking for the Matrix Principle.

Marysha Stephens
Belmont, NSW

Having done virtually no gym exercise for the first forty-eight years of my life, the Matrix system came as a great surprise to me. I had almost come to accept that as the years rolled on, my stomach would just keep getting

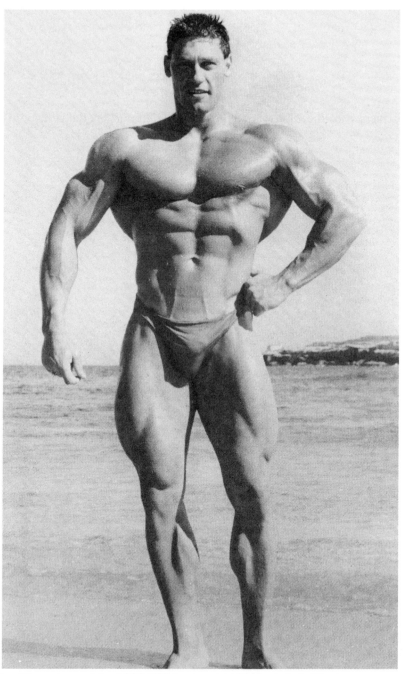

Ian Riley, winner of the 1988 IFBB heavyweight Mr Australasia title, is an outstanding example of the results achieved by Matrix training.

bigger. Within four months of Matrix training I gained four inches on my shoulders, added three inches to my chest and lost an incredible seven inches off my waist.

Ken Bargallie
Glendale, NSW

I had been training for several years off and on at my home and at gyms around the town, but I never really made much progress. The Matrix program made an amazing difference to my body within a few months. After a year of Matrix training I decided to compete in women's body-building. I won the Ms Sydney title and was runner-up in the Australian Superbowl of Bodybuilding. I wouldn't have believed it if I hadn't seen it.

Suzanne Kondraci
Wallsend, NSW

I had always felt in pretty good shape until my late-thirties came along. The next thing I knew my pants would no longer fit and I began to feel fat and flabby. Conventional gym training for a year or so did little for me. Then I tried Matrix training. Matrix has given me a new lease on my youth. In less than six months I have lost eight inches off my waist, put on five inches of muscle around my shoulders and four inches of solid muscle on my chest. My whole body has really changed, and I am actually looking forward to going to the beach this summer. I am a firm believer in the power of Matrix training.

Tom Cappon
Toronto, NSW

I am a cyclist but let myself get out of shape. Disgusted with my condition I took up gym training for at least a year to get back in shape. No matter how hard I tried, it seemed as if nothing was happening. Out of desperation I tried the Matrix system, and I have been utterly stunned by my progress. Within three months I lost ten pounds along with four inches off my waist. I gained four inches of muscle on my shoulders, over an inch on my arm, two inches on my thighs and three inches on my chest. Now, I actually seek the steep hills on my bicycle. The change in my body and in the way I feel is no less than incredible.

Geoffrey West
Tingira Heights, NSW

Part IV

Introductory Matrix routines

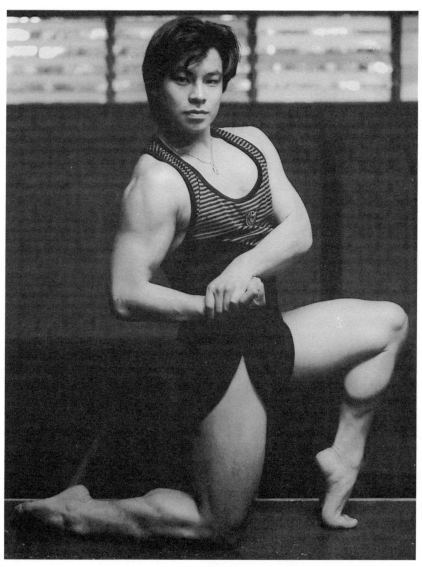

17 The introductory Matrix program

Of the several hundred Matrix exercises which have been devised, only a representative selection can be included in this book. Since our aim is to *introduce* the Matrix Principle to those who have not used it before, we have restricted ourselves to an outline of the introductory Matrix routines, leaving intermediate and advanced routines to a subsequent volume.

Seven body-parts are covered in these introductory routines. They are the chest, legs, biceps, triceps, deltoids, the lats and back, and the abdominal region. Those wishing to gain full advantage of Matrix exercise should work each body-part in Matrix mode at least once per week. As you become more advanced, each Matrix routine can be performed twice per week. Those who find a particular routine easy can perform it twice in the course of a workout with a pause of three minutes or so between the two runs. Those who find the above regimes too demanding, or whose time does not permit such a schedule, can reduce the frequency of Matrix training though obviously their progress will be slower and the results less spectacular.

Because of the high-intensity nature of this form of training, it is important to accustom oneself to Matrix workouts rather than rushing headlong into them. Naturally, before beginning this or any other exercise program, it is a sensible precaution to consult one's medical practitioner. The exercises described below are the 'standard' exercises which should soon be able to become the norm for those trainers who have a reasonable degree of strength and fitness. They may, however, be found difficult or even impossible to perform in 'standard' mode by beginners, older exercisers, or those who have done little weight-exercise in the past. These trainers are strongly advised not to give up on Matrix exercise because they find it too difficult in the early weeks. One, or all, of the following techniques should be used in order to accustom the body to the Matrix workout:

1 *Decrease the weight*   Matrix exercise is not based on the use of heavy weights, and can be performed quite effectively even with weights much lower than those indicated in the standard routines. If the weights mentioned below are found to be too heavy, decrease them by 5 kg (or 10 lb) until you reach a weight that is light enough to let you complete the required repetition pattern. For beginners or those who are less fit, even a broom stick, a length of pipe or an unloaded bar can be used to replace the normal barbell.

2 *Increase the pauses between sets*   This will increase your recuperation time and make the next exercise easier, though as you make progress you should move closer and closer to the short pauses indicated in the standard routines. The relative shortness of the pauses is an important aspect of Matrix training, and a key to its efficiency as a muscle-builder.

3 *Break up the sets*   As well as the pauses between sets, you can pause briefly within a set. As little as 5 seconds will sometimes enable you to recuperate sufficiently to complete the required set before passing on to the next.

If possible, the exercises and sequences should be performed in the order indicated in the routines below. For those who are exercising in a home gym, or who at least have their own weights and a few simple exercise machines, this should not present a problem. It will not always be a possibility, however, for those who do their workouts in a public or commercial gymnasium which has to be shared with other users. The machine or item of equipment which is required next in the sequence may not be available when the trainer needs it. When this is the case, the trainer will usually be able to stay with the machine or equipment that he or she has been using, and simply do a few more exercises in Matrix mode—using, say, a different grip or slightly different movement—until it is possible to move on to the equipment next required. If the normal rules of 'gym etiquette' prevail, the wait should not be unduly long.

The twelve different matrix techniques described below are incorporated into the programs which cover every body-part. Their combination provides the basis of substantial routines for trainers at every level of fitness.

The twelve Matrix techniques

1 *Conventional Matrix*

   5 full reps
   5 half-up
   5 half-down
   5 full reps

2 *Descending Matrix**

   7 full reps
   6 half-up
   5 half-down
   4 full reps

*The number of repetitions will vary depending upon the
exercise.

3 *Ascending Matrix**

   4 full reps
   5 half-up
   6 half-down
   7 full reps

*The number of repetitions will vary depending upon the
exercise.

4 *Matrix alternates*   Vid 3

   5 full reps
   +

1 half-up	1 half-up	1 half-up	1 half-up
1 half-down +	1 half-down +	1 half-down +	1 half-down
1 full rep	2 full reps	3 full reps	4 full reps

   +
   1 half-up
   1 half-down
   5 full reps

5 *Cumulative Matrix alternates*

1 full rep		2 full reps		3 half-up		4 half-up
1 half-up	+	2 half-up	+	3 half-down	+	4 half-down
1 half-down		2 half-down		4 full reps		5 full reps
		3 full reps				

6 *Matrix ladders*

5 full reps		1 rep ⅕ down
1 rep ⅕ up		1 rep ⅖ down
1 rep ⅖ up	+	1 rep ⅗ down
1 rep ⅗ up		1 rep ⅘ down
1 rep ⅘ up		1 full rep
1 full rep		5 full reps

7 *Cumulative Matrix ladders*

1 full rep		1 rep ⅕ down
1 rep ⅕ up		2 reps ⅖ down
2 reps ⅖ up	+	3 reps ⅗ down
3 reps ⅗ up		4 reps ⅘ down
4 reps ⅘ up		5 full reps
5 full reps		

8 *Ascending iso-Matrix*

5 full reps
1 rep half-up (holding weight in the half position for 1
  second)
1 rep half-up (hold for 2 seconds)
1 rep half-up (hold for 3 seconds)
1 rep half-up (hold for 4 seconds)
1 rep half-up (hold for 5 seconds)
1 full rep
  +
1 rep half-down (holding weight in the half position for 1
  second)
1 rep half-down (hold for 2 seconds)
1 rep half-down (hold for 3 seconds)
1 rep half-down (hold for 4 seconds)
1 rep half-down (hold for 5 seconds)
5 full reps

9   *Descending iso-Matrix*

5 full reps
1 rep half-up (holding weight in the half position for 5 seconds)
1 rep half-up (hold for 4 seconds)
1 rep half-up (hold for 3 seconds)
1 rep half-up (hold for 2 seconds)
1 rep half-up (hold for 1 second)
1 full rep
  +
1 rep half-down (holding weight in the half position for 5 seconds)
1 rep half-down (hold for 4 seconds)
1 rep half-down (hold for 3 seconds)
1 rep half-down (hold for 2 seconds)
1 rep half-down (hold for 1 second)
5 full reps

10   *Conventional iso-Matrix*

5 full reps
5 half-up (hold for 5 seconds*)
5 half-down (hold for 5 seconds)
5 full reps

* For beginners, hold for 3 seconds only.

11   *Cumulative iso-Matrix*

1 full rep
1 rep half-up (hold for 1 second)
2 reps half-up (hold for 2 seconds)
3 reps half-up (hold for 3 seconds)
4 reps half-up (hold for 4 seconds)
5 full reps
  +
1 rep half-down (hold for 1 second)
2 reps half-down (hold for 2 seconds)
3 reps half-down (hold for 3 seconds)
4 reps half-down (hold for 4 seconds)
5 full reps

12   *Mixed iso-Matrix*

5 full reps
3 reps half-up (hold for 3 seconds)
3 reps half-down (no holding)
3 reps half-up (no holding)
3 reps half-down (hold for 3 seconds)
5 full reps

Notes: For *half-up* movements, the weight should be raised to just above the half-way point of the movement. For *half-down* movements, the weight should be lowered to just below the half-way point of the movement. When a series of part reps is followed by full reps, ensure that you *complete* the part reps first; for example, at the end of a series of half-down bench presses followed by full presses, you should return the bar to the fully extended position on completion of the last half-down rep before lowering it to the chest to begin the full reps. When the instruction is to 'hold for 5 seconds', the intention is that the bar or dumbells will be held stationary at one or other of the above half positions or at a fractional position as in the case of the ladder Matrix.

Space does not permit a full description of every Matrix routine for each stage of each body-part. The following pages therefore consist of a brief description of each of the exercises used in the programs arranged by stages in ascending order of difficulty.

Stage I of each body-part Matrix is the beginner's stage, working progressively towards more advanced routines. Each stage should be completed as follows: once per week for the first four weeks; twice per week for the next three weeks. This makes a total of seven weeks' training for each stage, *before you move on to the next stage.*

Since there are seven stages, completion of the full Introductory Matrix Program takes 49 weeks, or almost one year. The remaining three weeks can be filled in by combining a high-level stage (e.g. V, VI or VII) with a lower-level stage (e.g. II, III or IV). Virtually any two stages can be combined, though combining in one workout two higher-level programs such as stages VI and VII would be extremely demanding.

Clinical tests have demonstrated that by following this Introductory Matrix Program faithfully for one year, you should in that period be able to gain the size and strength that would ordinarily take three to five years of conventional training to achieve.

Chest Matrix

Exercises used:

1 *Bench press*   Lie face up on the flat bench, positioning yourself so that your eyes are directly under the bar. Begin with a hand grip on the bar which is slightly wider than your shoulder width. As you press the bar, breathe in on the way down and exhale on the way up. Try not to let the bar bounce on the chest, as there is a delicate nerve centre in this area which can be damaged by improper technique. For Matrix training, vary the width of your grip with every bench-press exercise throughout every Matrix sequence.

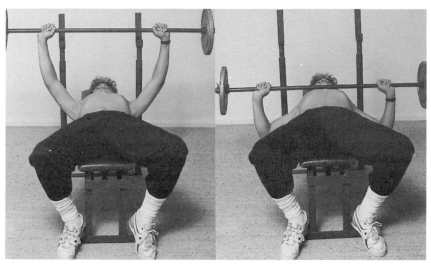

Bench Press up   down

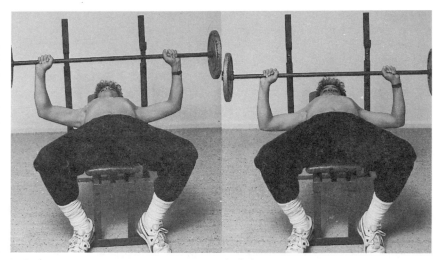

half-up   half-down

The starting weight should be about 40 per cent of your maximum single in this lift. (If you can bench press 90 kg (200 lb) for a single rep, begin with 40 per cent of that weight—90 kg × .40 = 36 kg or 80 lb). Use lighter weights if necessary, but increase the weight as you become stronger.

2 *Incline and decline press*   Performance is as for the flat bench press. If the bench is adjustable you can vary the angle of incline or decline with every set.

3 *Dumbbell flyes*   The weight should be about one-quarter of that used in the flat bench press. Lower the dumbbells slowly out to the side of the body, and bring them up in a wide arc. The elbows should be very slightly bent. For incline flyes, bring your arms up until they are almost straight overhead.

4 *Floor push-ups*   Lie face down on the floor, and place the palms of your hands on the floor at a comfortable distance from your shoulders. Your toes should be planted on the floor so that the ball of the foot just below the toes will, along with your hands, bear the weight of your body. Keeping your body rigid, press up from the floor until your arms have straightened. Lower your body to touch your chin to the floor for each repetition.

5 *Pec deck*   Begin by adjusting the height of the seat so that your shoulders are about 5 cm (2 or 3 in) below the top of the vertical pads. your forearms should be placed on the pads with your hands gripping the top of the pads (or the support bar, if there is one). Push against the pads until they touch in front of your torso. Hold this position for a second or two and release the pads slowly.

6 *Dips*   Grasping the handles of the dip bars tightly, press your body to arm's length. Keeping your chin tucked into your chest, and elbows out to the side of the body, lower your body slowly as far down as you can stretch, then raise yourself by pressing your body to arm's length. (Depending on your height and that of the dip bar, you may need a stool or bench to balance yourself as you mount the bar.)

Chest Matrix Schedule

Stage I

Sequence A

1 *Matrix Bench Press:*   5 full reps, 5 half-up, 5 half-down, 5 full reps
20 seconds pause

2 *Conventional Dumbbell Flyes:*   12 full reps
20 seconds pause

3 *Matrix Incline Press:*   5 full reps, 5 half-up, 5 half-down, 5 full reps
Pause three minutes

Sequence B

1 *Matrix Dumbbell Flyes:* 5 full reps, 5 half-up, 5 half-down, 5 full reps

20 seconds pause

2 *Conventional Incline Press:* 12 full reps

30 seconds pause

3 *Matrix Bench Press:* 5 full reps, 5 half-up, 5 half-down, 5 full reps

Pause three minutes

Sequence C

1 *Matrix Incline Press:* 5 full reps, 5 half-up, 5 half-down, 5 full reps

20 seconds pause

2 *Conventional Bench Press:* 12 full reps

40 seconds pause

3 *Matrix Dumbbell Flyes:* 5 full reps, 5 half-up, 5 half-down, 5 full reps

Finish

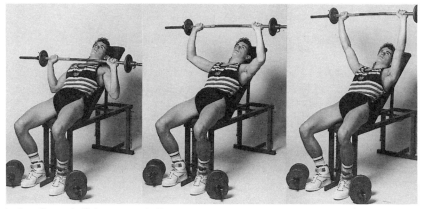

Incline Press half-down   half-up   up

Stage II

Sequence A

1 *Ascending Matrix Decline Bench Press:* 5 full reps, 6 half-up, 7 half-down, 8 full reps

20 seconds pause

2 *Conventional Pec Deck:* 15 full reps

30 seconds pause

3 *Matrix Floor Push-Ups:* 5 full reps, 5 half-up, 5 half-down, 5 full reps

Pause three minutes

Sequence B

1 *Ascending Matrix Pec Deck:*   4 full reps, 5 half-up, 6 half-down, 7 full reps

20 seconds pause

2 *Conventional Foor Push-Ups:*   15 full reps

30 seconds pause

3 *Matrix Decline Bench Press:*   5 full reps, 5 half-up, 5 half-down, 5 full reps

Pause three minutes

Sequence C

1 *Ascending Matrix Floor Push-Ups:*   4 full reps, 5 half-up, 6 half-down, 7 full reps

20 seconds pause

2 *Conventional Decline Bench Press:*   12 full reps

30 seconds pause

3 *Matrix Pec Deck:*   5 full reps, 5 half-up, 5 half-down, five full reps

Finish

Stage III

Sequence A

1 *Matrix Alternate Bench Press:*   5 full reps, 1 half-up, 1 half-down, 2 full reps, 1 half-up, 1 half-down, 3 full reps, 1 half-up, 1 half-down, 4 full reps, 1 half-up, 1 half-down, 5 full reps

20 seconds pause

2 *Conventional Dumbbell Flyes:*   12 full reps

30 seconds pause

3 *Ascending Matrix Incline Press:*   4 full reps, 5 half-up, 6 half-down, 7 full reps

Pause three minutes

Sequence B

1 *Matrix Alternate Dumbbell Flyes:*   5 full reps, 1 half-up, 1 half-down, 2 full reps, 1 half-up, 1 half-down, 3 full reps, 1 half-up, 1 half-down 4 full reps

30 seconds pause

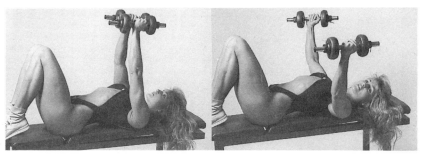

Dumbbell Flyes up   half-up

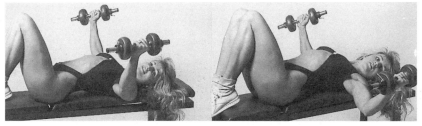

half-down   down

2 *Conventional Incline Press:* 10–12 full reps
30 seconds pause
3 *Ascending Matrix Bench Press:* 5 full reps, 6 half-up, 7 half-down, 8 full reps

Pause three minutes

Sequence C

1 *Matrix Alternate Incline Press:* 5 full reps, 1 half-up, 1 half-down, 2 full reps, 1 half-up, 1 half-down, 3 full reps, 1 half-up, 1 half-down, 4 full reps

30 seconds pause
2 *Conventional Bench Press:* 10–12 full reps
30 seconds pause
3 *Ascending Matrix Dumbbell Flyes* 4 full reps, 5 half-up, 6 half-down, 7 full reps

Finish

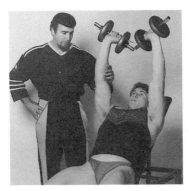 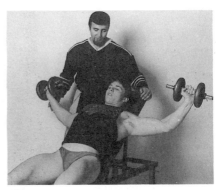

Incline Flyers   up   down

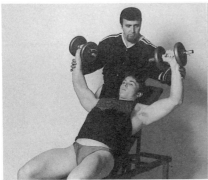 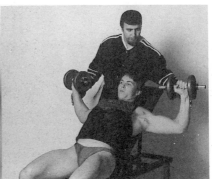

half-up   half-down

Stage IV

Sequence A

1   *Cumulative Matrix Alternate Decline Bench Press:*   1 full rep, 1
    half-up, 1 half-down, 2 full reps, 2 half-up, 2 half-down, 3 full reps,
    3 half-up, 3 half-down, 4 full reps, 4 half-up, 4 half-down, 5 full reps

    20 seconds pause

2   *Conventional Pec Deck:*   15 reps

    20 seconds pause

3   *Descending Matrix Floor Push-Ups:*   7 full reps, 6 half-up, 5 half-
    down, 4 full reps

    Pause two minutes

Sequence B

1   *Cumulative Matrix Pec Deck:*   1 full rep, 1 half-up, 1 half-down, 2
    full reps, 2 half-up, 2 half-down, 3 full reps, 3 half-up, 3 half-down,
    4 full reps, 4 half-up, 4 half-down, 5 full reps

    20 seconds pause

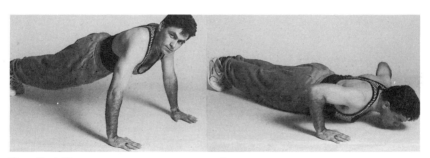

Floor Push-Ups   up   down

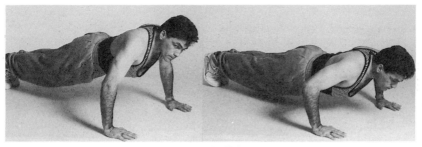

half-up   half-down

2   *Conventional Floor Push-Ups:*   15 reps

30 seconds pause

3   *Descending Matrix Decline Bench Press:*   7 full reps, 6 half-up, 5 half-down, 4 full reps

Pause three minutes

Sequence C

1   *Cumulative Matrix Floor Push-Ups:*   1 full rep, 1 half-up, 1 half-down, 2 full reps, 2 half-up, 2 half-down, 3 full reps, 3 half-up, 3 half-down, 4 full reps, 4 half-up, 4 half-down, 5 full reps

Finish

Stage V

Sequence A

1   *Ascending iso-Matrix Bench Press:*   5 full reps, 5 reps half-up (hold the first rep for 1 second, the second rep for 2 seconds and so on to a 5-second hold for the fifth rep), 5 reps half-down (hold the first rep for 1 second, the second rep for 2 seconds and so on to a 5-second hold for the fifth rep), 5 full reps

30 seconds pause

2   *Conventional Dumbbell Flyes:*   12 full reps

30 seconds pause

3   *Cumulative Matrix Alternate Incline Press:*   1 full rep, 1 half-up, 1 half-down, 2 full reps, 2 half-up, 2 half-down, 3 full reps, 3 half-up, 3 half-down, 4 full reps, 4 half-up, 4 half-down, 5 full reps

Pause three minutes

Sequence B

1   *Ascending iso-Matrix Dumbbell Flyes:*   3 full reps, 3 reps half-up (hold the first rep for 1 second, the second rep for 2 seconds and the third rep for 3 seconds), 3 half-down (hold each of the reps respectively from 1 to 3 seconds), 3 full reps

20 seconds pause

2   *Conventional Incline Press:*   10–12 full reps

20 seconds pause

3   *Cumulative Matrix Bench Press:*   1 full rep, 1 half-up, 1 half-down, 2 full reps, 2 half-up, 2 half-down, 3 full reps, 3 half-up, 3 half-down, 4 full reps

Pause three minutes

Sequence C

1   *Ascending iso-Matrix Incline Press:*   5 full reps, 5 reps half-up (hold each rep from 1 to 3 seconds progressively), 5 reps half-down (hold each rep from 1 to 5 seconds progressively), 5 full reps

30 seconds pause

2   *Conventional Bench Press:*   10–12 full reps

20 seconds pause

3   *Cumulative Matrix Dumbbell Flyes:*   1 full rep, 1 half-up, 1 half-down, 2 full reps, 2 half-up, 2 half-down, 3 full reps, 3 half-up, 3 half-down, 4 full reps

Finish

Stage VI

Sequence A

1   *Cumulative Matrix Decline Bench Press:*   1 full rep, 1 half-up, 1 half-down, 2 full reps, 2 half-up, 2 half-down, 3 full reps, 3 half-up, 3 half-down, 4 full reps, 4 half-up, 4 half-down, 5 full reps

20 seconds pause

2   *Conventional Pec Deck:*   15 full reps

20 seconds pause

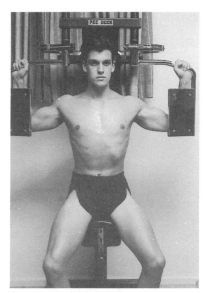

Pec Deck   down

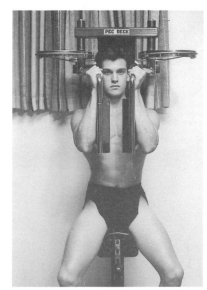

up

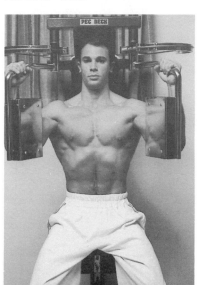

half-down

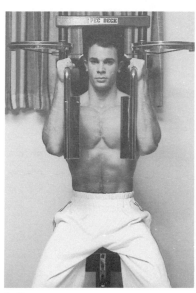

half-up

3   *Conventional iso-Matrix Floor Push-Ups:*   5 full reps, 5 half-up (hold each rep for 5 seconds), 5 half-down (hold each rep for 5 seconds), 5 full reps

Pause three minutes

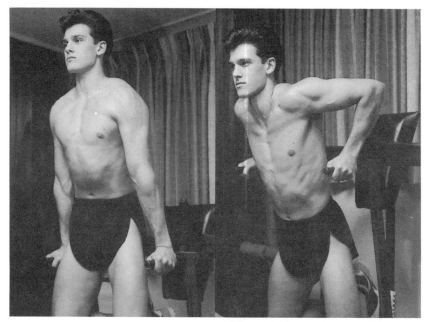

Dips   up   down

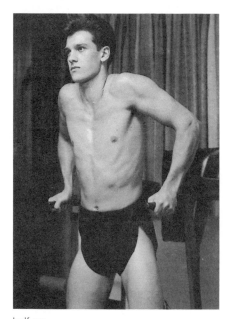

half-up

Sequence B

1 *Cumulative Matrix Pec Deck:*   1 full rep, 1 half-up, 1 half-down, 2 full reps, 2 half-up, 2 half-down, 3 full reps, 3 half-up, 3 half-down, 4 full reps

20 seconds pause

2 *Conventional Floor Push-Ups:*   15 full reps

30 seconds pause

3 *Conventional iso-Matrix Decline Bench Press:*   5 full reps, 5 half-up (hold each rep for 5 seconds), 5 half-down (hold each rep for 5 seconds), 5 full reps

Pause three minutes

Sequence C

1 *Cumulative Matrix Floor Push-Ups:*   1 full rep, 1 half-up, 1 half-down, 2 full reps, 2 half-up, 2 half-down, 3 full reps, 3 half-up, 3 half-down, 4 full reps

30 seconds pause

2 *Conventional Decline Bench Press:*   10–12 reps

30 seconds pause

3 *Conventional iso-Matrix Pec Deck:*   5 full reps, 5 half-up (hold each rep for 5 seconds), 5 half-down (hold each rep for 5 seconds), 5 full reps

Finish

Stage VII

Sequence A

1 *Cumulative iso-Matrix Bench Press:*   1 full rep, 1 half-up (hold for 1 second), 2 half-up (hold each rep for 2 seconds), continuing the cumulative pattern up to 5 reps (hold each rep for 5 seconds), 1 half-down (hold for 1 second), 2 half-down (hold each rep for 2 seconds), continuing the cumulative pattern up to 5 reps (hold each rep for 5 seconds), 5 full reps

30 seconds pause

2 *Conventional Dumbbell Flyes:*   12 full reps

30 seconds pause

3 *Cumulative Matrix Ladder Incline Press:*   1 full rep, 1 rep $1/5$-up, 2 reps $2/5$-up, 3 reps $3/5$-up, 4 reps $4/5$-up, 1 full rep, 1 rep $1/5$-down, 2 reps $2/5$-down, 3 reps $3/5$-down, 4 reps $4/5$-down, 5 full reps

Pause three minutes

Sequence B

1 *Cumulative iso-Matrix Dumbbell Flyes:*   1 full rep, 1 half-up (hold for 1 second), 2 half-up (hold each rep for 2 seconds), continuing the pattern to five reps (hold each rep for 5 seconds), 1 half-down (hold for 1 second), 2 half-down (hold each rep for 2 seconds), continuing the pattern to five reps (hold each rep for 5 seconds), 5 full reps

30 seconds pause

2 *Conventional Incline Press:*   12 full reps

30 seconds pause

3 *Cumulative Matrix Ladder Bench Press:*   1 full rep, 1 rep ⅕-up, 2 reps ⅖-up, 3 reps ⅗-up, 4 reps ⅘-up, 1 full rep, 1 rep ⅕-down, 2 reps ⅖-down, 3 reps ⅗-down, 4 reps ⅘-down, 5 full reps

Pause three minutes

Sequence C

1 *Cumulative iso-Matrix Incline Press:*   1 full rep, 1 half-up (hold for 1 second), 2 half-up (hold each rep for 2 seconds), continuing the pattern to five reps (hold each rep for 5 seconds), 1 half-down (hold for 1 second), 2 half-down (hold for 2 seconds), continuing the pattern to five reps (hold each rep for 5 seconds), 5 full reps

30 seconds pause

2 *Conventional Bench Press:*   12 full reps

30 seconds pause

3 *Cumulative Matrix Ladder Dumbbell Flyes:*   1 full rep, 1 rep ⅕-up, 2 reps ⅖-up, 3 reps ⅗-up, 4 reps ⅘-up, 1 full rep, 1 rep ⅕-down, 2 reps ⅖-down, 3 reps ⅗-down, 4 reps ⅘-down, 5 full reps

Finish

Thigh Matrix

Exercises used:

1 *Full squat*   With feet shoulder-width apart and toes turned slightly out, place the bar against the back of the shoulders and lift it off the rack. Bend the knees and inhale, lowering the body till the thighs are slightly lower than parallel to the floor. Push up again and exhale. The back must be kept straight, and the head held up. When viewed from the side, the line from the bar to the feet should remain vertical throughout the movement. (This exercise can also be performed on a squat machine.)

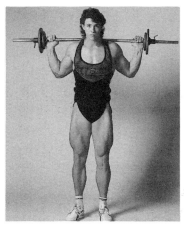

Full Squat   up

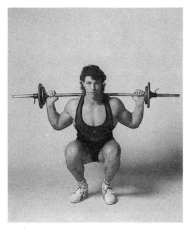

down

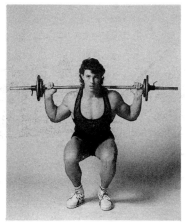

half-down

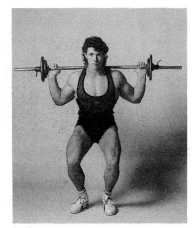

half-up

2   *Leg press*   Sit in the leg press machine, feet against the footplate. Bend the knees and lower the weight as far as possible. The knees should come back as close as possible to the shoulders. Press the weight back up slowly, being careful not to bounce it at the bottom of the movement.

3   *Leg extension*   Hook your feet under the pads on the machine, and extend your legs until they are locked out. Do not *lie* on the machine: sit upright and hold on to the seat with the hands. Slowly lower the weight again. Do not bounce the weight, or allow the buttocks to lift off the machine.

4   *Leg curl*   Lie face downward on the machine, hold on to the bench and hook your heels under the pads. Curl the legs slowly and release them slowly.

Thigh Matrix Schedule

Stage I

Sequence A

1   *Matrix Squat:*   5 full reps, 5 half-up, 5 half-down, 5 full reps

30 seconds pause

2   *Conventional Squat:*   12 full reps

30 seconds pause

3   *Matrix Leg Press:*   5 full reps, 5 half-up, 5 half-down, 5 full reps

30 seconds pause

4   *Conventional Leg Press:*   15 full reps

Three minutes pause

Sequence B

1   *Matrix Leg Press:*   5 full reps, 5 half-up, 5 half-down, 5 full reps

30 seconds pause

2   *Conventional Leg Press:*   15 full reps

30 seconds pause

3   *Matrix Squat:*   5 full reps, 5 half-up, 5 half-down, 5 full reps

30 seconds pause

4   *Conventional Squat:*   12 full reps

Finish

Stage II

Sequence A

1 *Ascending Matrix Leg Press:*   4 full reps, 5 half-up, 6 half-down, 7 full reps

30 seconds pause

2 *Descending Matrix Leg Press:*   7 full reps, 6 half-up, 5 half-down, 4 full reps

40 seconds pause

3 *Matrix Squat:*   5 full reps, 5 half-up, 5 half-down, 5 full reps

50 seconds pause

4 *Conventional Squat:*   12 full reps

Three minutes rest

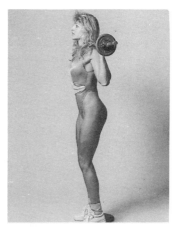

Full Squat   up

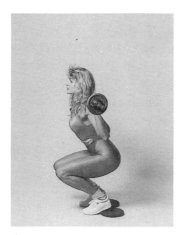

down

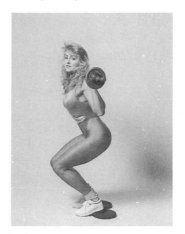

half-up

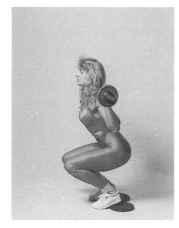

half-down

Sequence B

1 *Ascending Matrix Leg Press:*   4 full reps, 5 half-up, 6 half-down, 7 full reps

30 seconds pause

2 *Conventional Squat:*   12 full reps

40 seconds pause

3 *Descending Matrix Leg Press:*   7 full reps, 6 half-up, 5 half-down, 4 full reps

50 seconds pause

4 *Matrix Leg Press:*   5 full reps, 5 half-up, 5 half-down, 5 full reps

Finish

Stage III

Sequence A

1 *Matrix Squat:*   5 full reps, 5 half-up, 5 half-down, 5 full reps

30 seconds pause

2 *Conventional Leg Extensions:*   12–15 full reps

30 seconds pause

3 *Matrix Squat:*   5 full reps, 5 half-up, 5 half-down, 5 full reps

Three minutes pause

Sequence B

1 *Ascending Matrix Leg Press:*   4 full reps, 5 half-up, 6 half-down, 7 full reps

30 seconds pause

2 *Conventional Leg Extensions:*   12–15 full reps

30 seconds pause

3 *Ascending Matrix Leg Press:*   4 full reps, 5 half-up, 6 half-down, 7 full reps

Three minutes pause

Sequence C

1 *Matrix Alternate Squats:*   5 full reps, 1 half-up, 1 half-down, 1 full rep, 1 half-up, 1 half-down, 2 full reps, 1 half-up, 1 half-down, 3 full reps, 1 half-up, 1 half-down, 4 full reps, 1 half-up, 1 half-down, 5 full reps

30 seconds pause

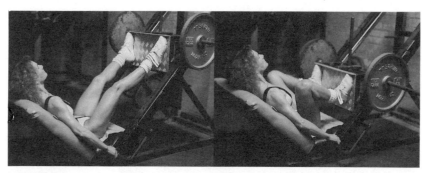

Leg Press   up   down

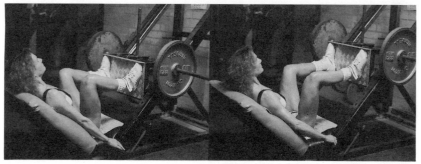

half-down   half-up

2 *Conventional Leg Extensions:*   12–15 full reps

40 seconds pause

3 *Matrix Alternate Leg Press:*   5 full reps, 1 half-up, 1 half-down, 1 full rep, 1 half-up, 1 half-down, 2 full reps, 1 half-up, 1 half-down, 3 full reps, 1 half-up, 1 half-down, 4 full reps, 1 half-up, 1 half-down, 5 full reps

Finish

Stage IV

Sequence A

1 *Cumulative Alternate Matrix Squat:*   1 full rep, 1 half-up, 1 half-down, 2 full reps, 2 half-up, 2 half-down, 3 full reps, 3 half-up, 3 half-down, 4 full reps, 4 half-up, 4 half-down, 5 full reps

30 seconds pause

2 *Conventional Leg Curls:*   12–15 full reps

40 seconds pause

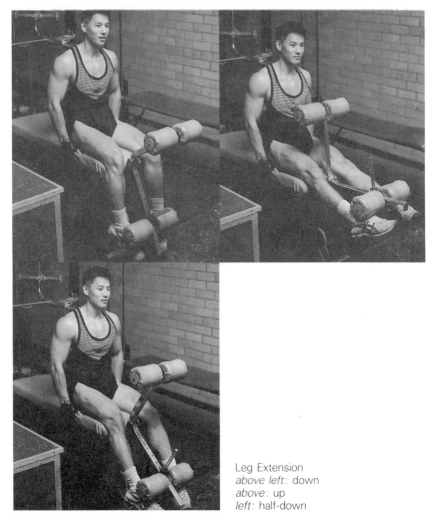

Leg Extension
above left: down
above: up
left: half-down

3 *Matrix Alternate Squat:* 5 full reps, 1 half-up, 1 half-down, 1 full rep, 1 half-up, 1 half-down, 2 full reps, 1 half-up, 1 half-down, 3 full reps, 1 half-up, 1 half-down, 4 full reps, 1 half-up, 1 half-down, 5 full reps

Three minutes pause

Sequence B

1 *Ascending Matrix Leg Press:* 4 full reps, 5 half-up, 6 half-down, 7 full reps

30 seconds pause

2 *Conventional Leg Curls:* 12–15 full reps

40 seconds pause

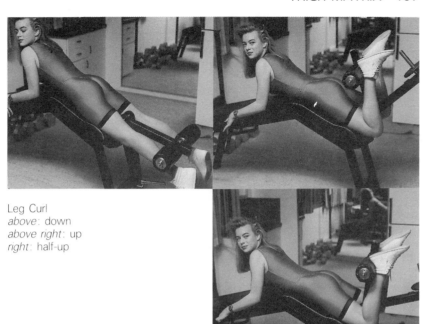

Leg Curl
above: down
above right: up
right: half-up

3   *Matrix Ladder Leg Press:*   5 full reps, 1 rep ⅕-up, 1 rep ⅖-up, 1 rep ⅗-up, 1 rep ⅘-up, 1 full rep, 1 rep ⅕-down, 1 rep ⅖-down, 1 rep ⅗-down, 1 rep ⅘-down, 1 full rep, 5 full reps

Three minutes pause

Sequence C

1   *Matrix Ladder Squat:*   5 full reps, 1 rep ⅕-up, 1 rep ⅖-up, 1 rep ⅗-up, 1 rep ⅘-up, 1 full rep, 1 rep ⅕-down, 1 rep ⅖-down, 1 rep ⅗-down, 1 rep ⅘ -down, 1 full rep, 5 full reps

30 seconds pause

2   *Conventional Leg Curls:*   12–15 reps

40 seconds pause

3   *Cumulative Alternate Matrix Leg Press:*   1 full rep, 1 half-up, 1 half-down, 2 full reps, 2 half-up, 2 half-down, 3 full reps, 3 half-up, 3 half-down, 4 full reps, 4 half-up, 4 half-down, 5 full reps

Finish

Stage V

Sequence A

1   *Iso-Matrix Squat:*   5 full reps, 5 half-up (hold for 5 seconds), 5

half-down (hold for 5 seconds), 5 full reps

30 seconds pause

2   *Matrix Alternate Leg Extensions:*   5 full reps, 1 half-up, 1 half-down, 1 full rep, 1 half-up, 1 half-down, 2 full reps, 1 half-up, 1 half-down, 3 full reps, 1 half-up, 1 half-down, 4 full reps, 1 half-up, 1 half-down, 5 full reps

30 seconds pause

3   *Matrix Ladder Leg Press:*   5 full reps, 1 rep $\frac{1}{5}$-up, 1 rep $\frac{2}{5}$-up, 1 rep $\frac{3}{5}$-up, 1 rep $\frac{4}{5}$-up, 1 full rep, 1 rep $\frac{1}{5}$-down, 1 rep $\frac{2}{5}$-down, 1 rep $\frac{3}{5}$-down, 1 rep $\frac{4}{5}$-down, 1 full rep, 5 full reps

Three minutes pause

Sequence B

1   *Iso-Matrix Leg Extensions:*   5 full reps, 5 half-up (hold for 5 seconds), 5 half-down (hold for 5 seconds), 5 full reps

30 seconds pause

2   *Matrix Alternate Leg Press:*   5 full reps, 1 half-up, 1 half-down, 1 full rep, 1 half-up, 1 half-down, 2 full reps, 1 half-up, 1 half-down, 3 full reps, 1 half-up, 1 half-down, 4 full reps, 1 half-up, 1 half-down, 5 full reps

30 seconds pause

3   *Matrix Ladder Squat:*   5 full reps, 1 rep $\frac{1}{5}$-up, 1 rep $\frac{2}{5}$-up, 1 rep $\frac{3}{5}$-up, 1 rep $\frac{4}{5}$-up, 1 full rep, 1 rep $\frac{1}{5}$-down, 1 rep $\frac{2}{5}$-down, 1 rep $\frac{3}{5}$-down, 1 rep $\frac{4}{5}$-down, 1 full rep, 5 full reps

Three minutes pause

Sequence C

1   *Iso-Matrix Leg Press:*   5 full reps, 5 half-up (hold for 5 seconds), 5 half-down (hold for 5 seconds), 5 full reps

30 seconds pause

2   *Matrix Alternate Squat:*   5 full reps, 1 half-up, 1 half-down, 1 full rep, 1 half-up, 1 half-down, 2 full reps, 1 half-up, 1 half-down, 3 full reps, 1 half-up, 1 half-down, 4 full reps, 1 half-up, 1 half down, 5 full reps

30 seconds pause

3   *Matrix Ladder Leg Extensions:*   5 full reps, 1 rep $\frac{1}{5}$-up, 1 rep $\frac{2}{5}$-up, 1 rep $\frac{3}{5}$-up, 1 rep $\frac{4}{5}$-up, 1 full rep, 1 rep $\frac{1}{5}$-down, 1 rep $\frac{2}{5}$-down, 1 rep $\frac{3}{5}$-down, 1 rep $\frac{4}{5}$-down, 1 full rep, 5 full reps

Finish

Stage VI

Sequence A

1   *Matrix Leg Press:*   5 full reps, 5 half-up, 5 half-down, 5 full reps

30 seconds pause

2   *Matrix Alternate Leg Press:*   5 full reps, 1 half-up, 1 half-down, 1 full rep, 1 half-up, 1 half-down, 2 full reps, 1 half-up, 1 half-down, 3 full reps, 1 half-up, 1 half-down, 4 full reps, 1 half-up, 1 half-down, 5 full reps

60 seconds pause

3   *Ascending Matrix Leg Press:*   4 full reps, 5 half-up, 6 half-down, 7 full reps

Three minutes pause

Sequence B

1   *Descending Matrix Squat:*   7 full reps, 6 half-up, 5 half-down, 4 full reps

30 seconds pause

2   *Matrix Alternate Squat:*   5 full reps, 1 half-up, 1 half-down, 1 full rep, 1 half-up, 1 half-down, 2 full reps, 1 half-up, 1 half-down, 3 full reps, 1 half-up, 1 half-down, 4 full reps, 1 half-up, 1 half-down, 5 full reps

60 seconds pause

3   *Matrix Squat:*   5 full reps, 5 half-up, 5 half-down, 5 full reps

Three minutes pause

Sequence C

1   *Ascending Matrix Leg Press:*   4 full reps, 5 half-up, 6 half-down, 7 full reps

30 seconds pause

2   *Descending Matrix Leg Press:*   7 full reps, 6 half-up, 5 half-down, 4 full reps

60 seconds pause

3   *Cumulative Matrix Alternate Leg Press:*   1 full rep, 1 half-up, 1 half-down, 2 full reps, 2 half-up, 2 half-down, 3 full reps, 3 half-up, 3 half-down, 4 full reps, 4 half-up, 4 half-down, 5 full reps

Finish

Stage VII

Sequence A

1   *Cumulative iso-Matrix Squat:*   1 full rep, 1 rep half-up (hold for 1

second), 2 reps half-up (hold for 2 seconds), 3 reps half-up (hold for 3 seconds), 4 reps half-up (hold for 4 seconds), 5 full reps, 1 rep half-down (hold for 1 second), 2 reps half-down (hold for 2 seconds), 3 reps half-down (hold for 3 seconds), 4 reps half-down (hold for 4 seconds), 5 full reps

30 seconds pause

2   *Cumulative Matrix Alternate Squat:*   1 full rep, 1 half-up, 1 half-down, 2 full reps, 2 half-up, 2 half-down, 3 full reps, 3 half-up, 3 half-down, 4 full reps, 4 half-up, 4 half-down, 5 full reps

50 seconds pause

3   *Matrix Ladder Squat:*   5 full reps, 1 rep ⅕-up, 1 rep ⅖-up, 1 rep ⅗-up, 1 rep ⅘-up, 1 full rep, 1 rep ⅕-down, 1 rep ⅖-down, 1 rep ⅗-down, 1 rep ⅘-down, 1 full rep, 5 full reps

Three minutes pause

Sequence B

1   *Ascending Matrix Leg Press:*   4 full reps, 5 half-up, 6 half-down, 7 full reps

30 seconds pause

2   *Mixed iso-Matrix Leg Press:*   5 full reps, 3 reps half-up (hold for 3 seconds), 3 reps half-down (no holding), 3 reps half-up (no holding), 3 reps half-down (hold for 3 seconds), 5 full reps

50 seconds pause

3   *Matrix Alternate Leg Press:*   5 full reps, 1 half-up, 1 half-down, 1 full rep, 1 half-up, 1 half-down, 2 full reps, 1 half-up, 1 half-down, 3 full reps, 1 half-up, 1 half-down, 4 full reps, 1 half-up, 1 half-down, 5 full reps

Three minutes pause

Sequence C

1   *Mixed iso-Matrix Squat:*   5 full reps, 3 reps half-up (hold for 3 seconds), 3 reps half-down (no holding), 3 reps half-up (no holding), 3 reps half-down (hold for 3 seconds), 5 full reps

30 seconds pause

2   *Descending Matrix Squat:*   7 full reps, 6 half-up, 5 half-down, 4 full reps

60 seconds pause

3   *Matrix Ladder Squat:*   5 full reps, 1 rep ⅕-up, 1 rep ⅖-up, 1 rep ⅗-up, 1 rep ⅘-up, 1 full rep, 1 rep ⅕-down, 1 rep ⅖-down, 1 rep ⅗-down, 1 rep ⅘-down, 1 full rep, 5 full reps

Finish

Biceps Matrix

Exercises used:

1 *Standing barbell curl*   Stand with feet slightly apart and grasp the bar with hands about shoulder-width apart. Curl the bar as you inhale, keeping the upper arm close to the body and as stationary as possible. Try not to sway the body. Slowly lower the bar as you exhale. Both positive and negative movements should be done in as wide an arc as possible. This exercise can be performed with a straight or E-Z curl bar, and the grip can be varied slightly from one set to another.

2 *Incline bench dumbbell curls*   Sit back on an incline bench, and curl the weights forward to shoulder level. Slowly lower the weights again. Do not swing the weights up at the end of each rep, but pause and raise them deliberately.

3 *Preacher bench curls*   Place the chest against the bench, which should be adjusted for height so that the upper arm lies along the bench rather than touching it only at the elbow. Curl the bar up slowly, and slowly lower it again. A straight or E-Z curl bar can be used. If you feel pain in the forearms, vary the grip or change the type of bar being used.

Biceps Matrix Schedule

Stage I

Sequence A

1 *Matrix Standing Barbell Curls:*   5 full reps, 5 half-up, 5 half-down, 5 full reps

30 seconds pause

2 *Conventional Incline Bench Dumbbell Curls:*   12 full reps

60 second pause

3 *Matrix Alternate Preacher Bench Curls*   5 full reps, 1 half-up, 1 half-down, 1 full rep, 1 half-up, 1 half-down, 2 full reps, 1 half-up, 1 half-down, 3 full reps, 1 half-up, 1 half-down, 4 full reps, 1 half-up, 1 half-down, 5 full reps

Three minutes pause

Sequence B

1 *Matrix Incline Bench Dumbbell Curls:*   5 full reps, 5 half-up, 5 half-down, 5 full reps

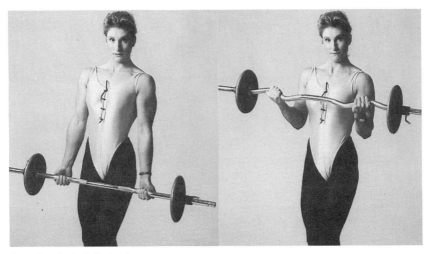

Standing Barbell Curl   down   up

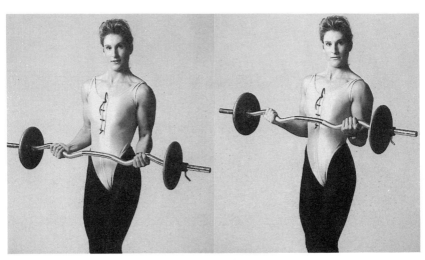

half-down   half-up

30 seconds pause

2 *Conventional Preacher Bench Curls:* 12 full reps

60 seconds pause

3 *Matrix Alternate Standing Barbell Curls:* 5 full reps, 1 half-up, 1 half-down, 1 full rep, 1 half-up, 1 half-down, 2 full reps, 1 half-up, 1 half-down, 3 full reps, 1 half-up, 1 half-down, 4 full reps, 1 half-up, 1 half-down, 5 full reps

Three minutes pause

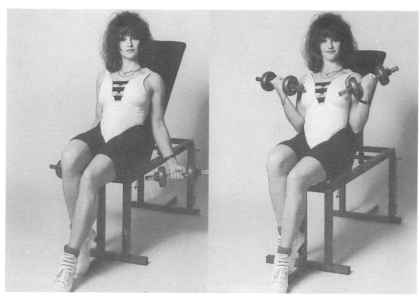

Incline Dumbbell Curl   down   up

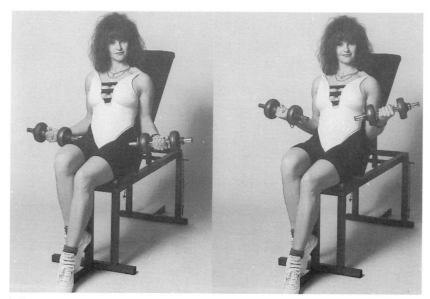

half-down   half-up

Sequence C

1 *Matrix Preacher Bench Curls:*   5 full reps, 5 half-up, 5 half-down,
   5 full reps

                    30 seconds pause

2 *Conventional Standing Barbell Curls:*   12 full reps

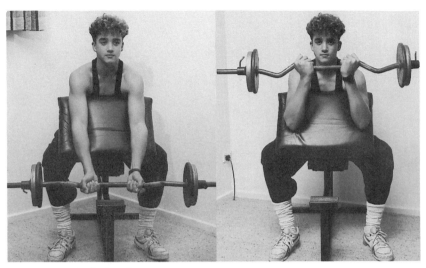

Preacher Bench Curls   down   up

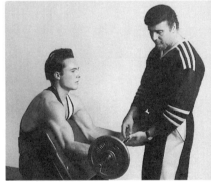

half-down   half-up

60 seconds pause

3 *Matrix Alternate Incline Bench Dumbbell Curls:* 5 full reps, 1 half-up, 1 half-down, 1 full rep, 1 half-up, 1 half-down, 2 full reps, 1 half-up, 1 half-down, 3 full reps, 1 half-up, 1 half-down, 4 full reps, 1 half-up, 1 half-down, 5 full reps

Finish

Stage II

Sequence A

1 *Matrix Alternate Preacher Bench Curls:* 5 full reps, 1 half-up, 1 half-down, 1 full rep, 1 half-up, 1 half-down, 2 full reps, 1 half-up,

1 half-down, 3 full reps, 1 half-up, 1 half-down, 4 full reps, 1 half-up, 1 half-down, 5 full reps

30 seconds pause

2   *Ascending Matrix Preacher Bench Curls:*   4 full reps, 5 half-up, 6 half-down, 7 full reps

60 seconds pause

3   *Conventional Preacher Bench Curls:*   12 full reps

Three minutes pause

Sequence B

1   *Cumulative Matrix Alternate Standing Barbell Curls:*   1 full rep, 1 half-up, 1 half-down, 2 full reps, 2 half-up, 2 half-down, 3 full reps, 3 half-up, 3 half-down, 4 full reps, 4 half-up, 4 half-down, 5 full reps

30 seconds pause

2   *Descending Matrix Standing Barbell Curls:*   7 full reps, 6 half-up, 5 half-down, 4 full reps

60 seconds pause

3   *Conventional Standing Barbell Curls:*   12 full reps

Three minutes pause

Sequence C

1   *Matrix Alternate Incline Bench Dumbbell Curls:*   5 full reps, 1 half-up, 1 half-down, 1 full rep, 1 half-up, 1 half-down, 2 full reps, 1 half-up, 1 half-down, 3 full reps, 1 half-up, 1 half-down, 4 full reps, 1 half-up, 1 half-down, 5 full reps

30 seconds pause

2   *Ascending Matrix Incline Bench Dumbbell Curls:*   4 full reps, 5 half-up, 6 half-down, 7 full reps

60 seconds pause

3   *Conventional Incline Bench Dumbbell Curls:*   12 full reps

Finish

Stage III

Sequence A

1   *Ascending Matrix Standing Barbell Curls:*   4 full reps, 5 half-up, 6 half-down, 7 full reps

30 seconds pause

2   *Descending Matrix Standing Barbell Curls:*   7 full reps, 6 half-up, 5 half-down, 4 full reps

60 seconds pause

3   *Matrix Alternate Standing Barbell Curls* 5 full reps, 1 half-up, 1 half-down, 1 full rep, 1 half-up, 1 half-down, 2 full reps, 1 half-up, 1 half-down, 3 full reps, 1 half-up, 1 half-down, 4 full reps, 1 half-up, 1 half-down, 5 full reps

Three minutes pause

Sequence B

1   *Cumulative Matrix Alternate Preacher Bench Curls:* 1 full rep, 1 half-up, 1 half-down, 2 full reps, 2 half-up, 2 half-down, 3 full reps, 3 half-up, 3 half-down, 4 full reps, 4 half-up, 4 half-down, 5 full reps

30 seconds pause

2   *Conventional Preacher Bench Curls:* 12 full reps

30 seconds pause

3   *Matrix Preacher Bench Curls:* 5 full reps, 5 half-up, 5 half-down, 5 full reps,

Three minutes pause

Sequence C

1   *Ascending Matrix Incline Bench Dumbbell Curls:* 4 full reps, 5 half-up, 6 half-down, 7 full reps

30 seconds pause

2   *Conventional Incline Bench Dumbbell Curls:*   5 full reps, 5 half-up, 5 half-down, 5 full reps

60 seconds pause

3   *Matrix Alternate Incline Bench Dumbbell Curls:*   5 full reps, 1 half-up, 1 half-down, 1 full rep, 1 half-up, 1 half-down, 2 full reps, 1 half-up, 1 half-down, 3 full reps, 1 half-up, 1 half-down, 4 full reps, 1 half-up, 1 half-down, 5 full reps

Finish

Stage IV

Sequence A

1   *Conventional iso-Matrix Standing Barbell Curls:* 5 full reps, 5 half-up (hold for 5 seconds), 5 half-down (hold for 5 seconds), 5 full reps

30 seconds pause

2   *Conventional Standing Barbell Curls:* 12 full reps

30 seconds pause

3   *Matrix Ladder Standing Barbell Curls:*   5 full reps, 1 rep ⅕-up, 1

rep ⅖-up, 1 rep ⅗-up, 1 rep ⅘-up, 1 full rep, 1 rep ⅕-down, 1 rep ⅖-down, 1 rep ⅗-down, 1 rep ⅘-down, 1 full rep, 5 full reps

Three minutes pause

Sequence B

1   *Cumulative iso-Matrix Preacher Bench Curls:*   1 full rep, 1 rep half-up (hold for 1 second), 2 reps half-up (hold for 2 seconds), 3 reps half-up (hold for 3 seconds), 4 reps half-up (hold for 4 seconds), 5 full reps, 1 rep half-down (hold for 1 second), 2 reps half-down (hold for 2 seconds), 3 reps half-down (hold for 3 seconds), 4 reps half-down (hold for 4 seconds), 5 full reps

30 seconds pause

2   *Conventional Preacher Bench Curls:*   12 full reps.

30 seconds pause

3   *Cumulative Matrix Alternate Curls:*   1 full rep, 1 half-up, 1 half-down, 2 full reps, 2 half-up, 2 half-down, 3 full reps, 3 half-up, 3 half-down, 4 full reps, 4 half-up, 4 half-down, 5 full reps

Three minutes pause

Sequence C

1   *Matrix Incline Bench Dumbbell Curls:*   5 full reps, 5 half-up, 5 half-down, 5 full reps

30 seconds pause

2   *Conventional Incline Bench Dumbbell Curls:*   10 full reps

30 seconds pause

3   *Conventional iso-Matrix Incline Bench Dumbbell Curls:*   5 full reps, 5 half-up (hold for 5 seconds), 5 half-down (hold for 5 seconds), 5 full reps

Finish

Stage V

Sequence A

1   *Cumulative iso-Matrix Standing Barbell Curls:*   1 full rep, 1 rep half-up (hold for 1 second), 2 reps half-up (hold for 2 seconds), 3 reps half-up (hold for 3 seconds), 4 reps half-up (hold for 4 seconds), 5 full reps, 1 rep half-down (hold for 1 second), 2 reps half-down (hold for 2 seconds), 3 reps half-down (hold for 3 seconds), 4 reps half-down (hold for 4 seconds), 5 full reps

20 seconds pause

2   *Cumulative Matrix Alternate Barbell Curls:*   1 full rep, 1 half-up, 1

half-down, 2 full reps, 2 half-up, 2 half-down, 3 full reps, 3 half-up, 3 half-down, 4 full reps, 4 half-up, 4 half-down, 5 full reps

30 seconds pause

3 *Conventional iso-Matrix Standing Barbell Curls:*   5 full reps, 5 half-up (hold for 5 seconds), 5 half-down (hold for 5 seconds), 5 full reps

Three minutes pause

Sequence B

1 *Cumulative iso-Matrix Incline Bench Dumbbell Curls:*   1 full rep, 1 rep half-up (hold for 1 second), 2 reps half-up (hold for 2 seconds), 3 reps half-up (hold for 3 seconds), 4 reps half-up (hold for 4 seconds), 5 full reps, 1 rep half-down (hold for 1 second), 2 reps half-down (hold for 2 seconds), 3 reps half-down (hold for 3 seconds), 4 reps half-down (hold for 4 seconds), 5 full reps

30 seconds pause

2 *Cumulative Matrix Alternate Incline Bench Dumbbell Curls:*   1 full rep, 1 half-up, 1 half-down, 2 full reps, 2 half-up, 2 half-down, 3 full reps, 3 half-up, 3 half-down, 4 full reps, 4 half-up, 4 half-down, 5 full reps

50 seconds pause

3 *Conventional iso-Matrix Incline Bench Dumbbell Curls:*   5 full reps, 5 half-up (hold for 5 seconds), 5 half-down (hold for 5 seconds), 5 full reps

Three minutes pause

Sequence C

1 *Cumulative iso-Matrix Preacher Bench Curls:*   1 full rep, 1 rep half-up (hold for 1 second), 2 reps half-up (hold for 2 seconds), 3 reps half-up (hold for 3 seconds), 4 reps half-up (hold for 4 seconds), 5 full reps, 1 rep half-down (hold for 1 second), 2 reps half-down (hold for 2 seconds), 3 reps half-down (hold for 3 seconds), 4 reps half-down (hold for 4 seconds), 5 full reps

30 seconds pause

2 *Cumulative Matrix Alternate Preacher Bench Curls:*   1 full rep, 1 half-up, 1 half-down, 2 full reps, 2 half-up, 2 half-down, 3 full reps, 3 half-dup, 3 half-down, 4 full reps, 4 half-dup, 4 half-down, 5 full reps

60 seconds pause

3 *Conventional iso-Matrix Preacher Bench Curls:*   5 full reps, 5 half-up (hold for 5 seconds), 5 half-down (hold for 5 seconds), 5 full reps

Finish

Stage VI

Sequence A

1   *Mixed iso-Matrix Preacher Bench Curls:*   5 full reps, 3 reps half-up (hold for 3 seconds), 3 reps half-down (no holding), 3 reps half-up (no holding), 3 reps half-down (hold for 3 seconds), 5 full reps

30 seconds pause

2   *Conventional Preacher Bench Curls:*   12 full reps

20 seconds pause

3   *Cumulative Matrix Ladder Preacher Bench Curls:*   1 full rep, 1 rep ⅕-up, 2 reps ⅖-up, 3 reps ⅗-up, 4 reps ⅘-up, 5 full reps, 1 rep ⅕-down, 2 reps ⅖-down, 3 reps ⅗-down, 4 reps ⅘-down, 5 full reps

30 seconds pause

4   *Matrix Alternate Preacher Bench Curls:*   5 full reps, 1 half-up, 1 half-down, 1 full rep, 1 half-up, 1 half-down, 2 full reps, 1 half-up, 1 half-down, 3 full reps, 1 half-up, 1 half-down, 4 full reps, 1 half-up, 1 half-down, 5 full reps

Three minutes pause

Sequence B

1   *Matrix Alternate Standing Barbell Curls:*   5 full reps, 1 half-up, 1 half-down, 1 full rep, 1 half-up, 1 half-down, 2 full reps, 1 half-up, 1 half-down, 3 full reps, 1 half-up, 1 half-down, 4 full reps, 1 half-up, 1 half-down, 5 full reps

30 seconds pause

2   *Cumulative Matrix Ladder Standing Barbell Curls:*   1 full rep, 1 rep ⅕-up, 2 reps ⅖-up, 3 reps ⅗-up, 4 reps ⅘-up, 5 full reps, 1 rep ⅕-down, 2 reps ⅖-down, 3 reps ⅗-down, 4 reps ⅘-down, 5 full reps

30 seconds pause

3   *Conventional Standing Barbell Curls:*   12 full reps

30 seconds pause

4   *Mixed iso-Matrix Standing Barbell Curls:*   5 full reps, 3 reps half-up (hold for 3 seconds), 3 reps half-down (no holding), 3 reps half-up (no holding), 3 reps half-down (hold for 3 seconds), 5 full reps *Finish*

Stage VII

Sequence A

1   *Ascending iso-Matrix Standing Barbell Curls:*   5 full reps, 1 rep half-up (hold for 1 second), 1 rep half-up (hold for 2 seconds), 1 rep half-up (hold for 3 seconds), 1 rep half-up (hold for 4 seconds), 1 rep half-up (hold for 5 seconds), 1 full rep, 1 rep half-down (hold for 1 second), 1 rep half-down (hold for 2 seconds), 1 rep half-down (hold

for 3 seconds), 1 rep half-down, (hold for 4 seconds), 1 rep half-down (hold for 5 seconds), 5 full reps

20 seconds pause

2   *Cumulative Matrix Alternate Standing Barbell Curls:*   1 full rep, 1 half-up, 1 half-down, 2 full reps, 2 half-up, 2 half-down, 3 full reps, 3 half-up, 3 half-down, 4 full reps, 4 half-up, 4 half-down, 5 full reps

20 seconds pause

3   *Descending iso-Matrix Standing Barbell Curls:*   5 full reps, 1 rep half-up (hold for 5 seconds), 1 rep half-up (hold for 4 seconds), 1 rep half-up (hold for 3 seconds), 1 rep half-up (hold for 2 seconds), 1 rep half-up (hold for 1 second), 1 full rep, 1 rep half-down (hold for 5 seconds), 1 rep half-down (hold for 4 seconds), 1 rep half-down (hold for 3 seconds), 1 rep half-down (hold for 2 seconds), 1 rep half-down (hold for 1 second), 5 full reps

Three minutes pause

Sequence B

1   *Cumulative Matrix Ladder Preacher Bench Curls:*   1 full rep, 1 rep ⅕-up, 2 reps ⅖-up, 3 reps ⅗-up, 4 reps ⅘-up, 5 full reps, 1 rep ⅕-down, 2 reps ⅖-down, 3 reps ⅗-down, 4 reps ⅘-down, 5 full reps

20 seconds pause

2   *Mixed iso-Matrix Preacher Bench Curls:*   5 full reps, 3 reps half-up (hold for 3 seconds), 3 reps half-down (no holding), 3 reps half-up (no holding), 3 reps half-down (hold for 3 seconds), 5 full reps

20 seconds pause

3   *Matrix Alternate Preacher Bench Curls:*   5 full reps, 1 half-up, 1 half-down, 1 full rep, 1 half-up, 1 half-down, 2 full reps, 1 half-up, 1 half-down, 3 full reps, 1 half-up, 1 half-down, 4 full reps, 1 half-up, 1 half-down, 5 full reps

Three minutes pause

Sequence C

1   *Matrix Incline Bench Dumbbell Curls:*   5 full reps, 5 half-up, 5 half-down, 5 full reps

20 seconds pause

2   *Conventional iso-Matrix Incline Bench Dumbbell Curls:*   5 full reps, 5 half-up (hold for 5 seconds), 5 half-down (hold for 5 seconds), 5 full reps

20 seconds pause

3   *Matrix Ladder Incline Bench Dumbbell Curls:*   5 full reps, 1 rep ⅕-up, 1 rep ⅖-up, 1 rep ⅗-up, 1 rep ⅘-up, 1 full rep, 1 rep ⅕-down, 1 rep ⅖-down, 1 rep ⅗-down, 1 rep ⅘-down, 1 full rep, 5 full reps

Finish

Triceps Matrix

Exercises used:

1 *Lying triceps press* Lie on a bench, with knees bent and feet resting on the bench. Grasp the bar with an overhand grip and press it up until the arms are locked out. The movement should end with the bar slightly behind the head. Without moving the elbows, slowly lower the bar towards the forehead then press it back to the starting position

2 *Standing triceps press* Hold a straight, E-Z curl or triceps bar with arms extended straight above the head. Slowly lower the bar as far as possible behind the head, moving the elbows as little as possible, then press it back up to the starting position.

3 *Triceps pushdowns* On the cable or lat machine, hold the straight or bent bar with an overhand grip, hands about 25 cm (10 in) apart. Press the bar down, keeping the upper arm stationary, and slowly let the bar come up again. Try to keep the body steady throughout the

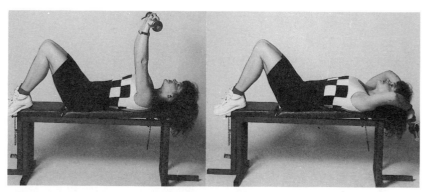

Lying Triceps Press   up   down

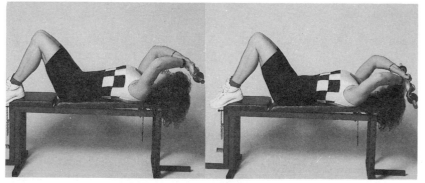

half-up   half-down

movement. Varying the width of the grip or the shape of the bar (or using a rope) hits the heads of the triceps in different ways.

4 *Dips*   (See also Chest Matrix). To maximise the effect on the triceps, try to keep the body perpendicular to the floor during the dip. Leaning forward engages the pecs more and thus reduces the isolation of the triceps.

Triceps Matrix Schedule

Stage I

Sequence A

1 *Matrix Lying Triceps Press:*   5 full reps, 5 half-up, 5 half-down, 5 full reps

30 seconds pause

2 *Conventional Standing Triceps Press:*   12 full reps

40 seconds pause

3 *Ascending Matrix Triceps Pushdowns:*   4 full reps, 5 half-up, 6 half-down, 7 full reps

Three minutes pause

Sequence B

1 *Matrix Standing Triceps Press:*   5 full reps, 5 half-up, 5 half-down, 5 full reps

30 seconds pause

2 *Conventional Triceps Pushdowns:*   12 full reps

40 seconds pause

3 *Ascending Matrix Lying Triceps Press:*   4 full reps, 5 half-up, 6 half-down, 7 full reps

Three minutes pause

Sequence C

1 *Matrix Triceps Pushdowns:*   5 full reps, 5 half-up, 5 half-down, 5 full reps

30 seconds pause

2 *Conventional Lying Triceps Press:*   12 full reps

40 seconds pause

3 *Ascending Matrix Standing Triceps Press:*   4 full reps, 5 half-up, 6 half-down, 7 full reps

Finish

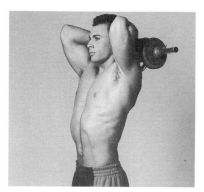 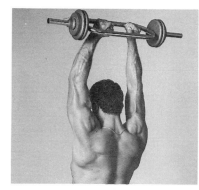

Standing Triceps Press   down   up

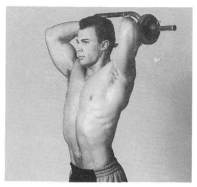 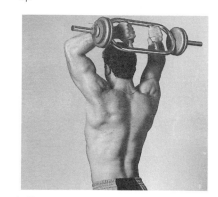

half-down   half-up

Stage II

Sequence A

1   *Ascending Matrix Triceps Pushdowns:*   4 full reps, 5 half-up, 6 half-down, 7 full reps

20 seconds pause

2   *Conventional Standing Triceps Press:*   12 full reps

30 seconds pause

3   *Matrix Alternate Lying Triceps Press:*   5 full reps, 1 half-up, 1 half-down, 1 full rep, 1 half-up, 1 half-down, 2 full reps, 1 half-up, 1 half-down, 3 full reps, 1 half-up, 1 half-down, 4 full reps, 1 half-up, 1 half-down, 5 full reps

Three minutes pause

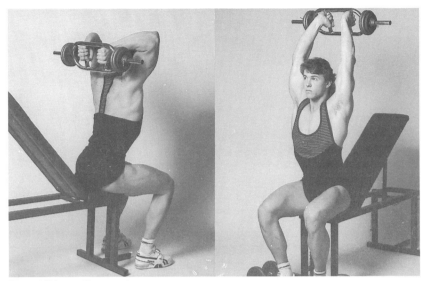

Seated Triceps Press   down   up

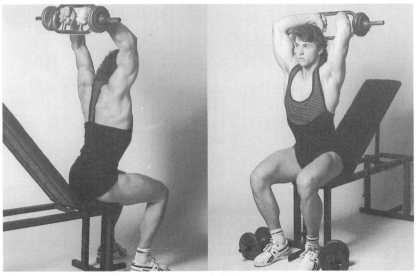

half-up   half-down

Sequence B

1   *Ascending Matrix Standing Triceps Press:*   4 full reps, 5 half-up, 6 half-down, 7 full reps

20 seconds pause

2   *Conventional Lying Triceps Press:*   12 full reps

30 seconds pause

3 *Matrix Alternate Triceps Pushdowns:* 5 full reps, 1 half-up, 1 half-down, 1 full rep, 1 half-up, 1 half-down, 2 full reps, 1 half-up, 1 half-down, 3 full reps, 1 half-up, 1 half-down, 4 full reps, 1 half-up, 1 half-down, 5 full reps

Three minutes pause

Sequence C

1 *Ascending Matrix Lying Triceps Press:* 4 full reps, 5 half-up, 6 half-down, 7 full reps

20 seconds pause

2 *Conventional Triceps Pushdowns:* 15 full reps

30 seconds pause

3 *Matrix Alternate Standing Triceps Press:* 5 full reps, 1 half-up, 1 half-down, 1 full rep, 1 half-up, 1 half-down, 2 full reps, 1 half-up, 1 half-down, 3 full reps, 1 half-up, 1 half-down, 4 full reps, 1 half-up, 1 half-down, 5 full reps

Finish

Stage III

Sequence A

1 *Cumulative Matrix Alternate Lying Triceps Press:* 1 full rep, 1 half-up, 1 half-down, 2 full reps, 2 half-up, 2 half-down, 3 full reps, 3 half-up, 3 half-down, 4 full reps, 4 half-up, 4 half-down, 5 full reps

20 seconds pause

2 *Conventional Dips:* 12 full reps or as many as possible up to 10

20 seconds pause

3 *Descending Matrix Standing Triceps Press:* 7 full reps, 6 half-up, 5 half-down, 4 full reps

Three minutes pause

Sequence B

1 *Cumulative Matrix Alternate Dips:* 1 full rep, 1 half-up, 1 half-down, 2 full reps, 2 half-up, 2 half-down, 3 full reps

20 seconds pause

2 *Conventional Standing Triceps Press:* 12 full reps

20 seconds pause

3 *Descending Matrix Lying Triceps Press:* 7 full reps, 6 half-up, 5 half-down, 4 full reps

Three minutes pause

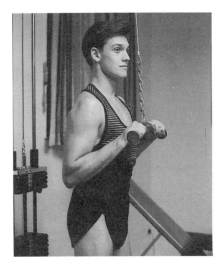

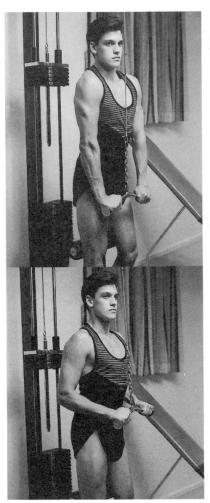

Triceps Pushdown
above: up
above right: down
right: half-down

Sequence C

1 *Cumulative Matrix Alternate Standing Triceps Press:* 1 full rep, 1 half-up, 1 half-down, 2 full reps, 2 half-up, 2 half-down, 3 full reps, 3 half-up, 3 half-down, 4 full reps, 4 half-up, 4 half-down, 5 full reps

20 seconds pause

2 *Conventional Lying Triceps Press:* 12 full reps

20 seconds pause

3 *Descending Matrix Dips:* 5 full reps, 4 half-up, 3 half-down, 2 full reps

Finish

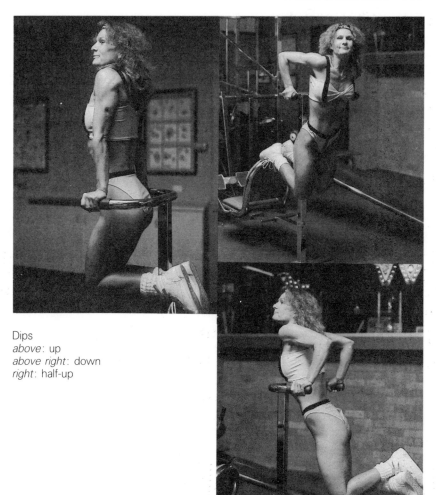

Dips
above: up
above right: down
right: half-up

Stage IV

Sequence A

1   *Conventional iso-Matrix Triceps Pushdowns:*   5 full reps, 5 half-up (hold for 5 seconds), 5 half-down (hold for 5 seconds), 5 full reps

20 seconds pause

2   *Conventional Standing Triceps Press:*   12 full reps

20 seconds pause

3   *Cumulative Matrix Alternate Lying Triceps Press:*   1 full rep, 1 half-up, 1 half-down, 2 full reps, 2 half-up, 2 half-down, 3 full reps, 3 half-up, 3 half-down, 4 full reps, 4 half-up, 4 half-down, 5 full reps

Two minutes pause

Sequence B

1   *Conventional iso-Matrix Standing Triceps Press:*   5 full reps, 5 half-up (hold for 5 seconds), 5 half-down (hold for 5 seconds), 5 full reps

20 seconds pause

2   *Conventional Lying Triceps Press:*   12 full reps

20 seconds pause

3   *Cumulative Matrix Triceps Pushdowns:*   1 full rep, 1 half-up, 1 half-down, 2 full reps, 2 half-up, 2 half-down, 3 full reps, 3 half-up, 3 half-down, 4 full reps, 4 half-up, 4 half-down, 5 full reps

Three minutes pause

Sequence C

1   *Conventional iso-Matrix Lying Triceps Press:*   5 full reps, 5 half-up (hold for 5 seconds), 5 half-down (hold for 5 seconds), 5 full reps

20 seconds pause

2   *Conventional Triceps Pushdowns:*   15 full reps

20 seconds pause

3   *Cumulative Matrix Standing Triceps Press:*   1 full rep, 1 half-up, 1 half-down, 2 full reps, 2 half-up, 2 half-down, 3 full reps, 3 half-up, 3 half-down, 4 full reps, 4 half-up, 4 half-down, 5 full reps

Finish

Stage V

Sequence A

1   *Matrix Standing Triceps Press:*   5 full reps, 5 half-up, 5 half-down, 5 full reps

20 seconds pause

2   *Cumulative Matrix Alternate Triceps Pushdowns:*   1 full rep, 1 half-up, 1 half-down, 2 full reps, 2 half-up, 2 half-down, 3 full reps, 3 half-up, 3 half-down, 4 full reps, 4 half-up, 4 half-down, 5 full reps

20 seconds pause

3   *Conventional Lying Triceps Press:*   12 full reps

Two minutes pause

Sequence B

1   *Matrix Triceps Pushdowns:*   5 full reps, 5 half-up, 5 half-down, 5 full reps

20 seconds pause

2 *Cumulative Matrix Lying Triceps Press:*   1 full rep, 1 half-up, 1 half-down, 2 full reps, 2 half-up, 2 half-down, 3 full reps, 3 half-up, 3 half-down, 4 full reps, 4 half-up, 4 half-down, 5 full reps

20 seconds pause

3 *Conventional Standing Triceps Press:*   12 full reps

Three minutes pause

Sequence C

1 *Matrix Lying Triceps Press:*   5 full reps, 5 half-up, 5 half-down, 5 full reps

20 seconds pause

2 *Cumulative Matrix Standing Triceps Press:*   1 full rep, 1 half-up, 1 half-down, 2 full reps, 2 half-up, 2 half-down, 3 full reps, 3 half-up, 3 half-down, 4 full reps, 4 half-up, 4 half-down, 5 full reps

20 seconds pause

3 *Conventional Triceps Pushdowns:*   15 full reps

Finish

Stage VI

Sequence A

1 *Matrix Ladder Triceps Pushdowns:*   5 full reps, 1 rep ⅕-up, 1 rep ⅖-up, 1 rep ⅗-up, 1 rep ⅘-up, 1 full rep, 1 rep ⅕-down, 1 rep ⅖-down, 1 rep ⅗-down, 1 rep ⅘-down, 1 full rep, 5 full reps

20 seconds pause

2 *Cumulative iso-Matrix Lying Triceps Press:*   1 full rep, 1 rep half-up (hold for 1 second), 2 reps half-up (hold for 2 seconds), 3 reps half-up (hold for 3 seconds), 4 reps half-up (hold for 4 seconds), 5 full reps, 1 rep half-down (hold for 1 second), 2 reps half-down (hold for 2 seconds), 3 reps half-down (hold for 3 seconds), 4 reps half-down (hold for 4 seconds), 5 full reps

20 seconds pause

3 *Matrix Alternate Standing Triceps Press:*   5 full reps, 1 half-up, 1 half-down, 1 full rep, 1 half-up, 1 half-down, 2 full reps, 1 half-up, 1 half-down, 3 full reps, 1 half-up, 1 half-down, 4 full reps, 1 half-up, 1 half-down, 5 full reps

Two minutes pause

Sequence B

1 *Matrix Ladder Lying Triceps Press:*   5 full reps, 1 rep ⅕-up, 1 rep ⅖-up, 1 rep ⅗-up, 1 rep ⅘-up, 1 full rep, 1 rep ⅕-down, 1 rep ⅖-down, 1 rep ⅗-down, 1 rep ⅘-down, 1 full rep, 5 full reps

20 seconds pause

2 *Cumulative iso-Matrix Standing Triceps Press:*   1 full rep, 1 rep half-up (hold for 1 second), 2 reps half-up (hold for 2 seconds), 3 reps half-up (hold for 3 seconds), 4 reps half-up (hold for 4 seconds), 5 full reps, 1 rep half-down (hold for 1 second), 2 reps half-down (hold for 2 seconds), 3 reps half-down (hold for 3 seconds), 4 reps half-down (hold for 4 seconds), 5 full reps

20 seconds pause

3 *Conventional Triceps Pushdowns:*   15 full reps

Two minutes pause

Sequence C

1 *Matrix Ladder Standing Triceps Press:*   5 full reps, 1 rep ⅕ up, 1 rep ⅖ up, 1 rep ⅗ up, 1 rep ⅘ up, 1 full rep, 1 rep ⅕ down, 1 rep ⅖ down, 1 rep ⅗ down, 1 rep ⅘ down, 1 full rep, 5 full reps

20 seconds pause

2 *Cumulative iso-Matrix Triceps Pushdowns:*   1 full rep, 1 rep half-up (hold for 1 second), 2 reps half-up (hold for 2 seconds), 3 reps half-up (hold for 3 seconds), 4 reps half-up (hold for 4 seconds), 5 full reps, 1 rep half-down (hold for 1 second), 2 reps half-down (hold for 2 seconds), 3 reps half-down (hold for 3 seconds), 4 reps half-down (hold for 4 seconds), 5 full reps

20 seconds pause

3 *Conventional Lying Triceps Press:*   12 full reps

Finish

Stage VII

Sequence A

1 *Mixed iso-Matrix Triceps Pushdowns:*   5 full reps, 3 reps half-up (hold for 3 seconds), 3 reps half-down (no holding), 3 reps half-up (no holding), 3 reps half-down (hold for 3 seconds), 5 full reps

20 seconds pause

2 *Cumulative Matrix Ladder Lying Triceps Press:*   1 full rep, 1 rep ⅕-up, 2 reps ⅖-up, 3 reps ⅗-up, 4 reps ⅘-up, 5 full reps, 1 rep ⅕-down, 2 reps ⅖-down, 3 reps ⅗-down, 4 reps ⅘-down, 5 full reps

20 seconds pause

3   *Cumulative Matrix Alternate Standing Triceps Press:*   1 full rep, 1 half-up, 1 half-down, 2 full reps, 2 half-up, 2 half-down, 3 full reps, 3 half-up, 3 half-down, 4 full reps, 4 half-up, 4 half-down, 5 full reps

Two minutes pause

Sequence B

1   *Mixed iso-Matrix Lying Triceps Press:*   5 full reps, 3 reps half-up (hold for 3 seconds), 3 reps half-down (no holding), 3 reps half-up (no holding), 3 reps half-down (hold for 3 seconds), 5 full reps

20 seconds pause

2   *Cumulative Matrix Ladder Standing Triceps Press:*   1 full rep, 1 rep ⅕-up, 2 reps ⅖-up, 3 reps ⅗-up, 4 reps ⅘-up, 5 full reps, 1 rep ⅕-down, 2 rep ⅖-down, 3 reps ⅗-down, 4 reps ⅘-down, 5 full reps

20 seconds pause

3   *Cumulative Matrix Alternate Triceps Pushdowns:*   1 full rep, 1 half-up, 1 half-down, 2 full reps, 2 half-up, 2 half-down, 3 full reps, 3 half-up, 3 half-down, 4 full reps, 4 half-up, 4 half-down, 5 full reps

Two minutes pause

Sequence C

1   *Mixed iso-Matrix Standing Triceps Press:*   5 full reps, 3 reps half-up (hold for 3 seconds), 3 reps half-down (no holding), 3 reps half-up (no holding), 3 reps half-down (hold for 3 seconds), 5 full reps

30 seconds pause

2   *Conventional Dips:*   as many consecutive reps as possible to exhaustion

30 seconds pause

3   *Cumulative Matrix Lying Triceps Press:*   1 full rep, 1 half-up, 1 half-down, 2 full reps, 2 half-up, 2 half-down, 3 full reps, 3 half-up, 3 half-down, 4 full reps, 4 half-up, 4 half-down, 5 full reps

Finish

Deltoid Matrix

Exercises used:

1 *Matrix roll presses*   Select a barbell of moderate to light weight. Using an overhand grip on the bar, hands spaced just wider than shoulder width, clear the weight to the top of the chest. From here, press the weight up to just above the half-way position and lower the bar down behind the neck until the bar gently touches the trapezius muscle at the base of the neck. Now return the bar to the original position on the chest by pressing it up to just above the half-way position and lowering it gently to the clavicle. When executed properly, the roll press movement will resemble the path of an arc or an upside down letter U. The completion of one repetition is marked by the passage of the bar from the front position on the chest to the traps in back of the neck *and return*. The repetition is not completed until the bar is returned to the position in front of the neck. If your shoulder muscles are tight, you may find it difficult at first to stretch comfortably in both directions. As you become accustomed to the exercise, it will become easier to perform. The exercise not only places the deltoids under continuous tension, but it forces co-operative contributions from all three heads of the deltoid to ensure maximum stimulation of the shoulder region.

2 *Dumbbell side laterals*   Take a dumbbell in each hand, holding them together in front of the body, Raise the arms to slightly above shoulder height, being careful not to swing the weights so as to use momentum. Turn the weights slightly forward as you raise them (as if pouring water from a bottle), and keep the elbows slightly unlocked. Lower the weights again slowly. This exercise can also be performed in a seated position, which helps keep the movement strict.

3 *Press behind the neck*   With the bar resting on the shoulders behind the neck (or lifted from the rack of a seated press bench), inhale as you press the weight straight up and exhale as you slowly lower it again. Keep the elbows as far back as possible throughout.

4 *Press in front of the neck*   The bar is held at the collarbone level, hands about shoulder width apart. Inhaling, lift the bar straight up till the arms are locked out, then lower it to the starting position as you exhale.

5 *Dumbbell front raises*   Stand with a dumbbell in each hand, held against the front of the thighs, or sit on a bench with the dumbbells held at arm's length beside you (the back of the hand facing forward). Lift the weights outwards straight in front of you, and up in a wide arc till they are higher than your head. Then slowly lower the weights in the same wide arc.

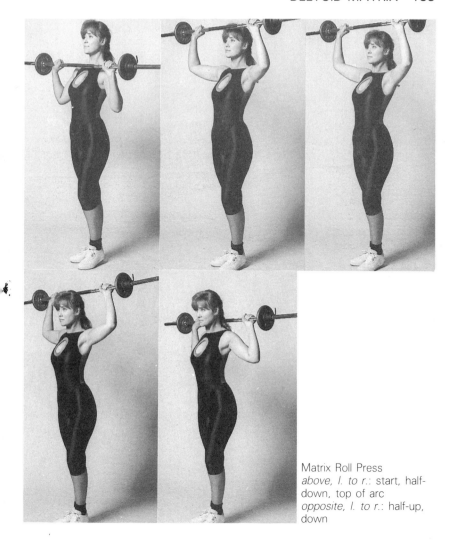

Matrix Roll Press
above, l. to r.: start, half-
down, top of arc
opposite, l. to r.: half-up,
down

6   *Upright rows*   Stand holding a barbell in front of your thighs with an overhand grip, hands a few centimetres apart. Inhaling, lift the bar until it almost touches the chin. Exhale as you lower the bar again, keeping the body as still as possible and not swinging or throwing the weight up.

Deltoid Matrix Schedule

Stage I

Sequence A

1   *Matrix Roll Press:*   5 full reps, 5 half-up, 5 half-down, 5 full reps
                        30 seconds pause

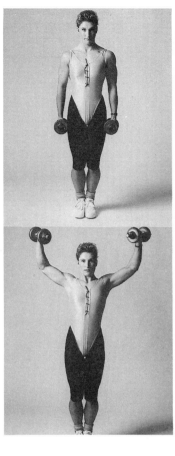
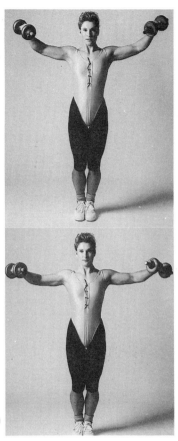

Dumbbell
Side
Laterals

down

up

half-up

half-down

2   *Conventional Dumbbell Side Laterals:*   12 full reps

30 seconds pause

3   *Behind the Neck Matrix Press:*   5 full reps, 5 half-up, 5 half-down, 5 full reps

Three minutes pause

Sequence B

1   *Matrix Roll Press:*   15 full reps

30 seconds pause

2   *Conventional Dumbbell Side Laterals:*   12 full reps

50 seconds pause

3   *In Front of the Neck Matrix Press:*   5 full reps, 5 half-up, 5 half-down, 5 full reps

Three minutes pause

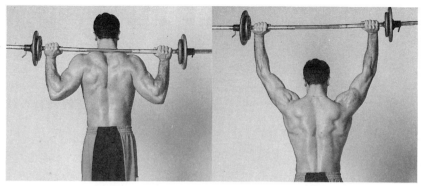

Press Behind the Neck   down   up

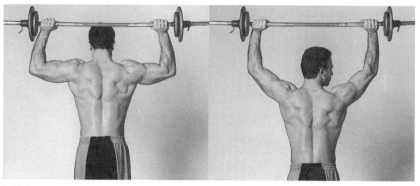

half-down   half-up

Sequence C

1 *Matrix Roll Press:* 15 full reps

                              30 seconds pause

2 *Conventional Dumbbell Side Laterals:* 12 full reps

                              60 seconds pause

3 *Matrix Roll Press:* 12–15 full reps

                              Finish

Stage II

Sequence A

1 *Matrix Roll Press:* 20 full reps

                              30 seconds pause

2 *Conventional Dumbbell Front Raises:* 12 full reps

                              40 seconds pause

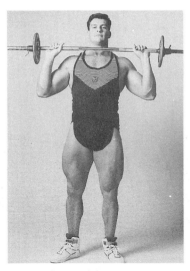 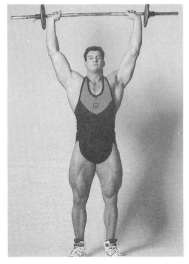

Press in Front of the Neck   down   up

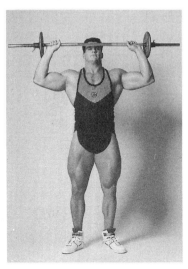 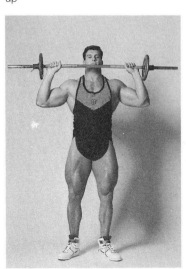

half-up   half-down

3 *Matrix Alternate Roll Press:*   15 roll presses, 1 rep half-up in front
   of the neck, 1 rep half-up behind the neck, 2 roll presses, 1 half-up
   in front, 1 half-up behind, 3 roll presses, 1 half-up in front, 1 half-up
   behind, 4 roll presses, 1 half-up in front, 1 half-up behind, 5 roll
   presses

Three minutes pause

Sequence B

1 *Matrix Roll Press:*   15 full reps

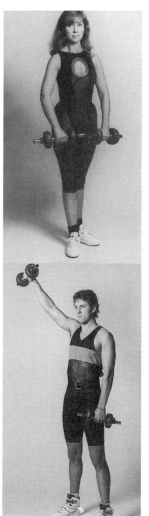

Dumbbell Front Raises

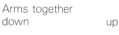

Arms together
down   up

Alternate arms
half-down   half-up

30 seconds pause

2   *Conventional Dumbbell Front Raises:* 12 full reps

50 seconds pause

3   *Matrix Alternate Roll Press:* 5 roll presses, 1 rep half-up in front of the neck, 1 rep half-up behind the neck, 2 roll presses, 1 half-up in front, 1 half-up behind, 3 roll presses, 1 half-up in front, 1 half-up behind, 4 roll presses, 1 half-up in front, 1 half-up behind, 5 roll presses.

Three minutes pause

Sequence C

1   *Matrix Roll Press:*   12 full reps

40 seconds pause

2   *Conventional Dumbbell Front Raises:* ·12 full reps

60 seconds pause

3   *Matrix Alternate Roll Press:*   5 roll presses, 1 rep half-up in front of the neck, 1 rep half-up behind the neck, 2 roll presses, 1 half-up in front, 1 half-up behind, 3 roll presses, 1 half-up in front, 1 half-up behind, 4 roll presses, 1 half-up in front, 1 half-up behind, 5 roll presses

Finish

Stage III

Sequence A

1   *Matrix Roll Press:*   20 full reps

20 seconds pause

2   *Conventional Dumbbell Side Laterals:*   12 full reps

30 seconds pause

3   *Cumulative Matrix Alternate Roll Press:*   1 rep half-up in front of the neck, 1 rep half-up behind the neck, 2 full reps, 2 reps half-up in front, 2 half-up behind, 3 full reps, 3 reps half-up in front, 3 half-up behind, 4 full reps, 4 reps half-up in front, 4 half-up behind, 5 roll presses

Three minutes pause

Sequence B

1   *Matrix Roll Press:*   15 full reps

30 seconds pause

2   *Conventional Dumbbell Side Laterals:*   10–12 full reps

40 seconds pause

3   *Cumulative Matrix Alternate Roll Press:*   1 rep half-up in front of the neck, 1 rep half-up behind the neck, 2 full reps, 2 reps half-up in front, 2 half-up behind, 3 full reps, 3 reps half-up in front, 3 half-up behind, 4 full reps, 4 reps half-up in front, 4 half-up behind, 5 roll presses

Three minutes pause

Sequence C

1   *Matrix Roll Press:*   12–15 full reps

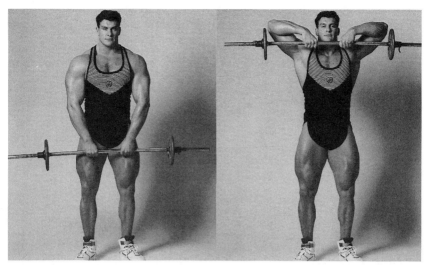

Upright Rows   down   up

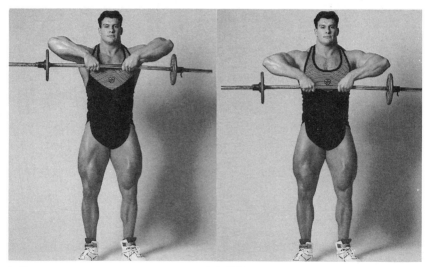

half-up   half-down

40 seconds pause

2   *Conventional Dumbbell Side Laterals:*   10–12 reps

50 seconds pause

3   *Cumulative Matrix Alternate Roll Press:*   1 rep half-up in front of the neck, 1 rep half-up behind the neck, 2 full reps, 2 reps half-up in front , 2 half-up behind, 3 full reps, 3 reps half-up in front, 3 half-up behind, 4 full reps, 4 reps half-up in front, 4 half-up behind, 5 roll presses

Finish

Stage IV

Sequence A

1   *Matrix Alternate Roll Press:*   15 roll presses, 1 rep half-up in front of the neck, 1 rep half-up behind the neck, 2 roll presses, 1 half-up in front, 1 half-up behind, 3 roll presses, 1 half-up in front, 1 half-up behind, 4 roll presses, 1 half-up in front, 1 half-up behind, 5 roll presses

20 seconds pause

2   *Conventional Upright Rows:*   15 full reps

30 seconds pause

3   *Conventional Half-Up iso-Matrix Roll Press:*   5 roll presses, 5 reps half-up in front of the neck (hold for 5 seconds), 5 reps half-up behind the neck (hold for 5 seconds), 5 roll presses

Three minutes pause

Sequence B

1   *Matrix Alternate Roll Press:*   15 roll presses, 1 rep half-up in front of the neck, 1 rep half-up behind the neck, 2 roll presses, 1 half-up in front, 1 half-up behind, 3 roll presses, 1 half-up in front, 1 half-up behind, 4 roll presses, 1 half-up in front, 1 half-up behind, 5 roll presses

20 seconds pause

2   *Conventional Upright Rows:*   15 full reps

40 seconds pause

3   *Conventional Half-Down iso-Matrix Roll Press:*   5 roll presses, 5 reps from the top position half-down in front of the neck (hold for 5 seconds), 5 reps from the top position half-down behind the neck (hold for 5 seconds), 5 roll presses

Three minutes pause

Sequence C

1   *Matrix Alternate Roll Press:*   15 roll presses, 1 rep half-up in front of the neck, 1 rep half-up behind the neck, 2 roll presses, 1 half-up in front, 1 half-up behind, 3 roll presses, 1 half-up in front, 1 half-up behind, 4 roll presses, 1 half-up in front, 1 half-up behind, 5 roll presses

30 seconds pause

2   *Conventional Upright Rows:*   12–15 full reps

30 seconds pause

3   *Conventional Half-Up iso-Matrix Roll Press:*   5 roll presses, 5 reps half-up in front of the neck (hold for 5 seconds), 5 reps half-up behind the neck (hold for 5 seconds), 5 roll presses

Finish

Stage V

Sequence A

1   *Cumulative Matrix Alternate Roll Press:*   1 rep half-up in front of the neck, 1 rep half-up behind the neck, 2 full reps, 2 reps half-up in front, 2 half-up behind, 3 full reps, 3 reps half-up in front, 3 half-up behind, 4 full reps, 4 reps half-up in front, 4 half-up behind, 5 roll presses

20 seconds pause

2   *Matrix Upright Rows:*   5 full reps, 5 half-up, 5 half-down, 5 full reps

30 seconds pause

3   *Matrix Ladder Roll Press:*   5 roll presses, 1 rep $\frac{1}{5}$-up in front of neck, 1 rep $\frac{2}{5}$-up, 1 rep $\frac{3}{5}$-up, 1 rep $\frac{4}{5}$-up, 1 full rep, 1 rep $\frac{1}{5}$-up behind the neck, 1 rep $\frac{2}{5}$-up behind the neck, 1 rep $\frac{3}{5}$-up behind the neck, 1 rep $\frac{4}{5}$-up behind the neck, 1 full rep, 5 roll presses

Three minutes pause

Sequence B

1   *Cumulative Matrix Alternate Roll Press:*   1 rep half-up in front of the neck, 1 rep half-up behind the neck, 2 full reps, 2 reps half-up in front, 2 half-up behind, 3 full reps, 3 reps half-up in front, 3 half-up behind, 4 full reps, 4 reps half-up in front, 4 half-up behind, 5 roll presses

20 seconds pause

2   *Conventional Upright Rows:*   15 full reps

20 seconds pause

3   *Matrix Ladder Roll Press:*   5 roll presses, 1 rep $\frac{1}{5}$-up in front of neck, 1 rep $\frac{2}{5}$-up, 1 rep $\frac{3}{5}$-up, 1 rep $\frac{4}{5}$-up, 1 full rep, 1 rep $\frac{1}{5}$-up behind the neck, 1 rep $\frac{2}{5}$-up behind the neck, 1 rep $\frac{3}{5}$-up behind the neck, 1 rep $\frac{4}{5}$-up behind the neck, 1 full rep, 5 roll presses

Three minutes pause

Sequence C

1   *Cumulative Matrix Alternate Roll Press:*   1 rep half-up in front of the neck, 1 rep half-up behind the neck, 2 full reps, 2 reps half-up in front, 2 half-up behind, 3 full reps, 3 reps half-up in front, 3 half-up

behind, 4 full reps, 4 reps half-up in front, 4 half-up behind, 5 roll presses

20 seconds pause

2   *Matrix Upright Rows:*   5 full reps, 5 half-up, 5 half-down, 5 full reps

30 seconds pause

3   *Matrix Ladder Roll Press:*   5 roll presses, 1 rep $\frac{1}{5}$-up in front of neck, 1 rep $\frac{2}{5}$-up, 1 rep $\frac{3}{5}$-up, 1 rep $\frac{4}{5}$-up, 1 full rep, 1 rep $\frac{1}{5}$-up behind the neck, 1 rep $\frac{2}{5}$-up behind the neck, 1 rep $\frac{3}{5}$-up behind the neck, 1 rep $\frac{4}{5}$-up behind the neck, 1 full rep, 5 roll presses

Finish

Stage VI

Sequence A

1   *Conventional Half-Up iso-Matrix Roll Press:*   5 roll presses, 5 reps half-up in front of the neck (hold for 5 seconds), 5 reps half-up behind the neck (hold for 5 seconds), 5 roll presses

20 seconds pause

2   *Matrix Dumbbell Side Laterals:*   5 full reps, 5 half-up, 5 half-down, 5 full reps

30 seconds pause

3   *Mixed iso-Matrix Behind the Neck Press:*   5 roll presses, 3 reps half-up (hold for 3 seconds), 3 reps half-down (no holding), 3 reps half-up (no holding), 3 reps half-down (hold for 3 seconds), 5 roll presses

Three minutes pause

Sequence B

1   *Conventional Half-Down iso-Matrix Roll Press:*   5 roll presses, 5 reps from the top position half-down in front of the neck (hold for 5 seconds), 5 reps from the top position half-down behind the neck (hold for 5 seconds), 5 roll presses

20 seconds pause

2   *Matrix Alternate Dumbbell Side Laterals:*   5 full reps, 5 half-up, 5 half-down, 5 full reps

30 seconds pause

3   *Mixed iso-Matrix In Front of the Neck Press:*   5 roll presses, 3 reps half-up (hold for 3 seconds), 3 reps half-down (no holding), 3 reps half-up (no holding), 3 reps half-down (hold for 3 seconds), 5 roll presses

Three minutes pause

Sequence C

1 *Cumulative Matrix Alternate Roll Press:* 1 rep half-up in front of
   the neck, 1 rep half-up behind the neck, 2 full reps, 2 reps half-up in
   front, 2 half-up behind, 3 full reps, 3 reps half-up in front, 3 half-up
   behind, 4 full reps, 4 reps half-up in front, 4 half-up behind, 5 roll
   presses

20 seconds pause

2 *Matrix Ladder Dumbbell Side Laterals:* 5 full reps, 5 half-up, 5
   half-down, 5 full reps

20 seconds pause

3 *Matrix Roll Press:* 20 full reps

Finish

Stage VII

Sequence A

1 *Matrix Roll Press:* 20 full reps

20 seconds pause

2 *Matrix Alternate Roll Press:* 15 roll presses, 1 rep half-up in front
   of the neck, 1 rep half-up behind the neck, 2 roll presses, 1 half-up
   in front, 1 half-up behind, 3 roll presses, 1 half-up in front, 1 half-up
   behind, 4 roll presses, 1 half-up in front, 1 half-up behind, 5 roll
   presses

20 seconds pause

3 *Matrix Ladder Roll Press:* 5 roll presses, 1 rep $\frac{1}{5}$-up in front of
   neck, 1 rep $\frac{2}{5}$-up, 1 rep $\frac{3}{5}$-up, 1 rep $\frac{4}{5}$-up, 1 full rep, 1 rep $\frac{1}{5}$-up
   behind the neck, 1 rep $\frac{2}{5}$-up behind the neck, 1 rep $\frac{3}{5}$-up behind the
   neck, 1 rep $\frac{4}{5}$-up behind the neck, 1 full rep, 5 roll presses

One minute pause

Sequence B

1 *Matrix Upright Rows:* 5 full reps, 5 half-up, 5 half-down, 5 full reps

20 seconds pause

2 *Matrix Alternate Upright Rows:* 5 full reps, 1 half-up, 1 half-down,
   1 full rep, 1 half-up, 1 half-down, 2 full reps, 1 half-up, 1 half-down,
   3 full reps, 1 half-up, 1 half-down, 4 full reps, 1 half-up, 1 half-down,
   5 full reps

30 seconds pause

3 *Cumulative iso-Matrix Upright Rows:* 1 full rep, 1 rep half-up (hold
   for 1 second), 2 reps half-up (hold for 2 seconds), 3 reps half-up (hold
   for 3 seconds), 4 reps half-up (hold for 4 seconds), 5 full reps, 1 rep

half-down (hold for 1 second), 2 reps half-down (hold for 2 seconds), 3 reps half-down (hold for 3 seconds), 4 reps half-down (hold for 4 seconds), 5 full reps

Three minutes pause

Sequence C

1   *Cumulative Alternate Matrix Roll Press:*   1 rep half-up in front of the neck, 1 rep half-up behind the neck, 2 full reps, 2 reps half-up in front, 2 half-up behind, 3 full reps, 3 reps half-up in front, 3 half-up behind, 4 full reps, 4 reps half-up in front, 4 half-up behind, 5 roll presses

20 seconds pause

2   *Conventional Half-Up iso-Matrix Roll Press:*   5 roll presses, 5 reps half-up in front of the neck (hold for 5 seconds), 5 reps half-up behind the neck (hold for 5 seconds), 5 roll presses

20 seconds pause

3   *Matrix Ladder Roll Press:*   5 roll presses, 1 rep $\frac{1}{5}$-up in front of neck, 1 rep $\frac{2}{5}$-up, 1 rep $\frac{3}{5}$-up, 1 rep $\frac{4}{5}$-up, 1 full rep, 1 rep $\frac{1}{5}$-up behind the neck, 1 rep $\frac{2}{5}$-up behind the neck, 1 rep $\frac{3}{5}$-up behind the neck, 1 rep $\frac{4}{5}$-up behind the neck, 1 full rep, 5 roll presses

Finish

Lats and Back Matrix

Exercises used:

1 *Bent-over rows*   With feet a few centimetres apart and knees slightly bent, bend forward at the waist and lift the bar a few centimetres off the floor, keeping the back straight and letting the bar hang at arm's length. Inhale as you lift the bar upwards until it touches the chest or upper abdomen, consciously trying to use the lats as much as possible (rather than the arms). Exhaling, slowly lower the bar again to the starting position. Alternatively, this exercise can be performed lying face-down on a suitably designed incline bench.

2 *Chin-ups in front of the neck*   Grasp the bar with an overhand grip and pull yourself up as you inhale, trying to touch the bar with the top of the chest. Briefly hold at the top of the movement and lower yourself to the starting position as you exhale. The grip should be as wide as is comfortable.

3 *Chin-ups behind the neck*   As for the above, except that you pull yourself up until the back of the neck touches the bar. Chins should be performed as strictly as possible, trying not to kick up with the legs for momentum.

4 *Lat machine pulldowns*   With knees anchored by the support on the lat machine, grasp the bar with a fairly wide grip and as you inhale, pull the bar down till it reaches the back of the neck (or top of the chest). Slowly extend the arms as you exhale, to return the bar to the starting position.

5 *Stiff-legged deadlifts*   Place a barbell on the floor in front of you, bend forward from the waist with back straight, and grasp the bar with an overhand grip. Straighten up and come to a standing position, pulling the shoulders back and arching the spine. Keep the legs straight and knees locked. Lower the bar again by bending forward from the waist.

6 *Bent-arm pullovers.*   Lie on the bench, with the bar on the floor behind the head. Grasp the bar and (inhaling) raise it with bent arms, just over the head, to the chest. As you exhale, slowly lower the bar back to just above the starting position, not letting it touch the floor.

7 *Hyperextensions*   Face down on the hyperextension bench, heels locked under the supports, bend forward as far as possible with hands clasped in front of the chest or behind the head. Slowly straighten up again until the torso is just above parallel to the floor. Do not come up too far and arch the back.

Bent-Over Rows
on bench

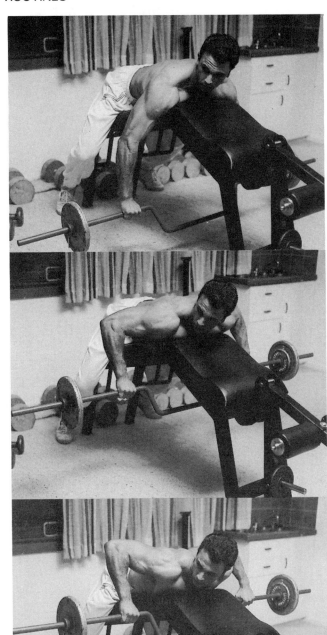

down

half-up

up

Bent-over Rows

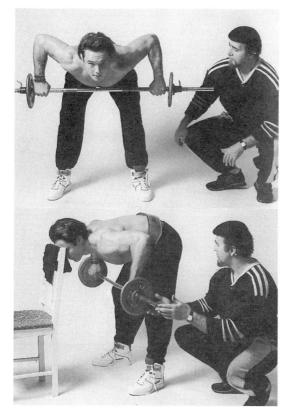

up

half-up

Lats and Back Matrix Schedule

Stage I

Sequence A

1   *Matrix Bent-Over Rows:*   5 full reps, 5 half-up, 5 half-down, 5 full reps

   30 seconds pause

2   *Conventional Chin-Ups (in front of neck):*   As many as possible up to 15 reps

   60 seconds pause

3   *Matrix Alternate Lat Machine Pulldowns:*   5 full reps, 1 half-up, 1 half-down, 1 full rep, 1 half-up, 1 half-down, 2 full reps, 1 half-up, 1 half-down, 3 full reps, 1 half-up, 1 half-down, 4 full reps, 1 half-up, 1 half-down, 5 full reps

   Two minutes pause

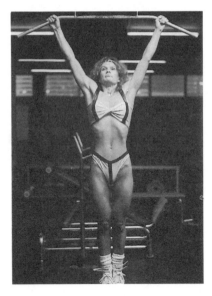

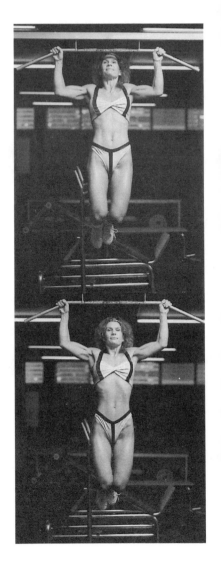

Chin-Ups in Front of Neck
above: down
above right: half-up
right: half-down

Sequence B

1 *Matrix Lat Machine Pulldowns:* 5 full reps, 5 half-up, 5 half-down, 5 full reps

30 seconds pause

2 *Conventional Chin-Ups:* As many as possible up to 15 reps

60 seconds pause

3 *Matrix Alternate Bent-Over Rows:* 5 full reps, 1 half-up, 1 half-down, 1 full rep, 1 half-up, 1 half-down, 2 full reps, 1 half-up, 1 half-down, 3 full reps, 1 half-up, 1 half-down, 4 full reps, 1 half-up, 1 half-down, 5 full reps

Three minutes pause

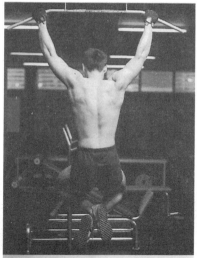

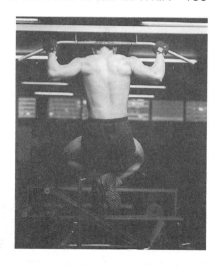

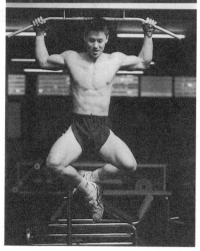

Chin-Ups behind Neck
above left: down
above: up
left: half-up

Sequence C

1 *Matrix Bent-Over Rows:* 5 full reps, 5 half-up, 5 half-down, 5 full reps

30 seconds pause

2 *Conventional Chin-Ups:* As many as possible up to 15 reps

60 seconds pause

3 *Matrix Alternate Lat Machine Pulldowns:* 5 full reps, 1 half-up, 1 half-down, 1 full rep, 1 half-up, 1 half-down, 2 full reps, 1 half-up, 1 half-down, 3 full reps, 1 half-up, 1 half-down, 4 full reps, 1 half-up, 1 half-down, 5 full reps

Finish

Stage II

Sequence A

1   *Matrix Alternate Lat Machine Pulldowns:*   5 full reps, 1 half-up, 1 half-down, 1 full rep, 1 half-up, 1 half-down, 2 full reps, 1 half-up, 1 half-down, 3 full reps, 1 half-up, 1 half-down, 4 full reps, 1 half-up, 1 half-down, 5 full reps

20 seconds pause

2   *Conventional Stiff-Legged Deadlift:*   12 full reps

20 seconds pause

3   *Cumulative Matrix Alternate Bent-Over Rows:*   1 full rep, 1 half-up, 1 half-down, 2 full reps, 2 half-up, 2 half-down, 3 full reps, 3 half-up, 3 half-down, 4 full reps, 4 half-up, 4 half-down, 5 full reps

Two minutes pause

Sequence B

1   *Matrix Alternate Bent-Over Rows:*   5 full reps, 1 half-up, 1 half-down, 1 full rep, 1 half-up, 1 half-down, 2 full reps, 1 half-up, 1 half-down, 3 full reps, 1 half-up, 1 half-down, 4 full reps, 1 half-up, 1 half-down, 5 full reps

20 seconds pause

2   *Conventional Chin-Ups:*   As many as possible up to 15 reps

50 seconds pause

3   *Cumulative Matrix Alternate Lat Machine Pulldowns:*   1 full rep, 1 half-up, 1 half-down, 2 full reps, 2 half-up, 2 half-down, 3 full reps, 3 half-up, 3 half-down, 4 full reps, 4 half-up, 4 half-down, 5 full reps

Three minutes pause

Sequence C

1   *Matrix Alternate Lat Machine Pulldowns:*   5 full reps, 1 half-up, 1 half-down, 1 full rep, 1 half-up, 1 half-down, 2 full reps, 1 half-up, 1 half-down, 3 full reps, 1 half-up, 1 half-down, 4 full reps, 1 half-up, 1 half-down, 5 full reps

20 seconds pause

2   *Conventional Stiff-Legged Deadlifts:*   12 full reps

50 seconds pause

3   *Cumulative Matrix Alternate Bent-Over Rows:*   1 full rep, 1 half-up, 1 half-down, 2 full reps, 2 half-up, 2 half-down, 3 full reps, 3 half-up, 3 half-down, 4 full reps, 4 half-up, 4 half-down, 5 full reps

Finish

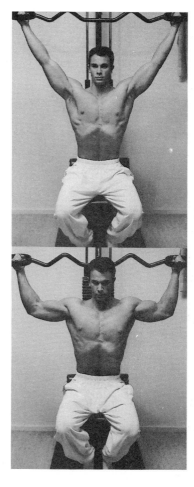

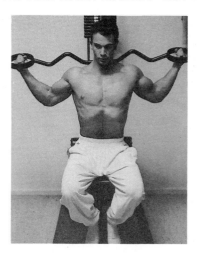

Lat Machine
Pulldowns behind
Neck
above left: up
above: down
left: half-down

Stage III

Sequence A

1 *Cumulative Matrix Alternate Bent-Over Rows:* 1 full rep, 1 half-up,
   1 half-down, 2 full reps, 2 half-up, 2 half-down, 3 full reps, 3 half-up,
   3 half-down, 4 full reps, 4 half-up, 4 half-down, 5 full reps

20 seconds pause

2 *Conventional Bent-Arm Pullovers:* 15 full reps

20 seconds pause

3 *Matrix Ladder Lat Machine Pulldowns:* 5 full reps, 1 rep $\frac{1}{5}$-up, 1
   rep $\frac{2}{5}$-up, 1 rep $\frac{3}{5}$-up, 1 rep $\frac{4}{5}$-up, 1 full rep, 1 rep $\frac{1}{5}$-down, 1 rep
   $\frac{2}{5}$-down, 1 rep $\frac{3}{5}$-down, 1 rep $\frac{4}{5}$-down, 1 full rep, 5 full reps

Two minutes pause

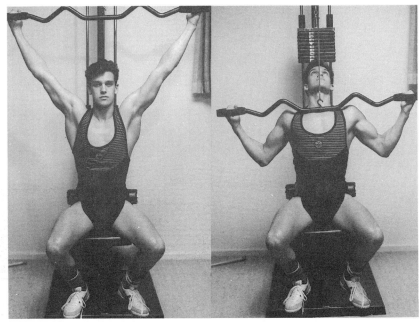

Lat Machine Pulldowns in front of Neck   up   down

Sequence B

1   *Cumulative Matrix Lat Machine Pulldowns:*   1 full rep, 1 half-up, 1 half-down, 2 full reps, 2 half-up, 2 half-down, 3 full reps, 3 half-up, 3 half-down, 4 full reps, 4 half-up, 4 half-down, 5 full reps

20 seconds pause

2   *Conventional Stiff-Legged Deadlifts:*   12 full reps

20 seconds pause

3   *Matrix Ladder Bent-Over Rows:*   5 full reps, 1 rep ⅕-up, 1 rep ⅖-up, 1 rep ⅗-up, 1 rep ⅘-up, 1 full rep, 1 rep ⅕-down, 1 rep ⅖-down, 1 rep ⅗-down, 1 rep ⅘-down, 1 full rep, 5 full reps

Three minutes pause

Sequence C

1   *Cumulative Matrix Bent-Over Rows:*   1 full rep, 1 half-up, 1 half-down, 2 full reps, 2 half-up, 2 half-down, 3 full reps, 3 half-up, 3 half-down, 4 full reps, 4 half-up, 4 half-down, 5 full reps

20 seconds pause

2   *Conventional Bent-Arm Pullovers:*   15 full reps

20 seconds pause

3   *Matrix Ladder Lat Machine Pulldowns:*   5 full reps, 1 rep ⅕-up, 1 rep ⅖-up, 1 rep ⅗-up, 1 rep ⅘-up, 1 full rep, 1 rep ⅕-down, 1 rep

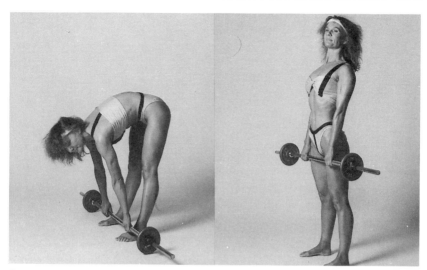

Stiff-legged Deadlift   down   up

⅖-down, 1 rep ⅗-down, 1 rep ⅘-down, 1 full rep, 5 full reps
Finish

Stage IV

Sequence A

1   *Cumulative Matrix Ladder Lat Machine Pulldowns:*   1 full rep, 1
    rep ⅕-up, 2 reps ⅖-up, 3 reps ⅗-up, 4 reps ⅘-up, 5 full reps, 1 rep
    ⅕-down, 2 reps ⅖-down, 3 reps ⅗-down, 4 reps ⅘-down, 5 full reps
                        20 seconds pause
2   *Matrix Hyperextensions:*   5 full reps, 5 half-up, 5 half-down, 5 full
    reps
                        20 seconds pause
3   *Ascending Matrix Bent-Over Rows:*   4 full reps, 5 half-up, 6 half-
    down, 7 full reps
                        Two minutes pause

Sequence B

1   *Cumulative Matrix Ladder Bent-Over Rows:*   1 full rep, 1 rep ⅕-up,
    2 reps ⅖-up, 3 reps ⅗-up, 4 reps ⅘-up, 5 full reps, 1 rep ⅕-down,
    2 reps ⅖-down, 3 reps ⅗-down, 4 reps ⅘-down, 5 full reps
                        20 seconds pause

2   *Matrix Alternate Hyperextensions:*   5 full reps, 1 half-up, 1 half-down, 1 full rep, 1 half-up, 1 half-down, 2 full reps, 1 half-up, 1 half-down, 3 full reps, 1 half-up, 1 half-down, 4 full reps, 1 half-up, 1 half-down, 5 full reps

20 seconds pause

3   *Ascending Matrix Lat Machine Pulldowns:*   4 full reps, 5 half-up, 6 half-down, 7 full reps

Two minutes pause

Sequence B

1   *Cumulative Matrix Ladder Lat Machine Pulldowns:*   1 full rep, 1 rep $\frac{1}{5}$-up, 2 reps $\frac{2}{5}$-up, 3 reps $\frac{3}{5}$-up, 4 reps $\frac{4}{5}$-up, 5 full reps, 1 rep $\frac{1}{5}$-down, 2 reps $\frac{2}{5}$-down, 3 reps $\frac{3}{5}$-down, 4 reps $\frac{4}{5}$-down, 5 full reps

20 seconds pause

2   *Cumulative Matrix Alternate Hyperextensions:*   1 full rep, 1 half-up, 1 half-down, 2 full reps, 2 half-up, 2 half-down, 3 full reps, 3 half-up, 3 half-down, 4 full reps, 4 half-up, 4 half-down, 5 full reps

20 seconds pause

3   *Ascending Matrix Bent-Over-Rows:*   4 full reps, 5 half-up, 6 half-down, 7 full reps

Finish

Stage V

Sequence A

1   *Ascending iso-Matrix Bent-Over Rows:*   5 full reps, 1 rep half-up (hold for 1 second), 1 rep half-up (hold for 2 seconds), 1 rep half-up (hold for 3 seconds), 1 rep half-up (hold for 4 seconds), 1 rep half-up (hold for 5 seconds), 1 full rep, 1 rep half-down (hold for 1 second), 1 rep half-down (hold for 2 seconds), 1 rep half-down (hold for 3 seconds), 1 rep half-down (hold for 4 seconds), 1 rep half-down (hold for 5 seconds), 5 full reps

20 seconds pause

2   *Conventional Chin-Ups:*   As many as possible up to 15 reps

20 seconds pause

3   *Cumulative Matrix Alternate Lat Machine Pulldowns:*   1 full rep, 1 half-up, 1 half-down, 2 full reps, 2 half-up, 2 half-down, 3 full reps, 3 half-up, 3 half-down, 4 full reps, 4 half-up, 4 half-down, 5 full reps

Two minutes pause

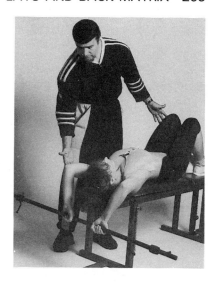

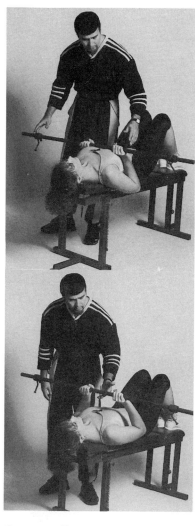

Bent-Arm Pullovers
above left: up
above: down
left: half-up

Sequence B

1 *Ascending iso-Matrix Lat Machine Pulldowns:* 5 full reps, 1 rep half-up (hold for 1 second), 1 rep half-up (hold for 2 seconds), 1 rep half-up (hold for 3 seconds), 1 rep half-up (hold for 4 seconds), 1 rep half-up (hold for 5 seconds), 1 full rep, 1 rep half-down (hold for 1 second), 1 rep half-down (hold for 2 seconds), 1 rep half-down (hold for 3 seconds), 1 rep half-down (hold for 4 seconds), 1 rep half-down (hold for 5 seconds), 5 full reps

30 seconds pause

2 *Conventional Chin-Ups:* As many as possible up to 15 reps

20 seconds pause

Hyperextensions

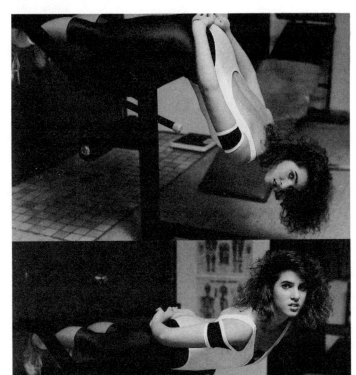

down

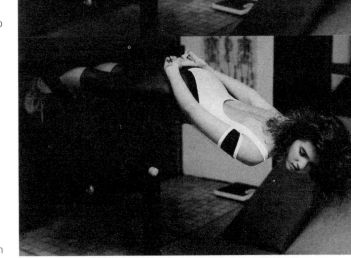

up

half-down

3 *Cumulative Matrix Alternate Bent-Over Rows:*   1 full rep, 1 half-up, 1 half-down, 2 full reps, 2 half-up, 2 half-down, 3 full reps, 3 half-up, 3 half-down, 4 full reps, 4 half-up, 4 half-down, 5 full reps

Two minutes pause

Sequence C

1 *Ascending iso-Matrix Bent-Over Rows:*   5 full reps, 1 rep half-up (hold for 1 second), 1 rep half-up (hold for 2 seconds), 1 rep half-up (hold for 3 seconds), 1 rep half-up (hold for 4 seconds), 1 rep half-up (hold for 5 seconds), 1 full rep, 1 rep half-down (hold for 1 second), 1 rep half-down (hold for 2 seconds), 1 rep half-down (hold for 3 seconds), 1 rep half-down (hold for 4 seconds), 1 rep half-down (hold for 5 seconds), 5 full reps

30 seconds pause

2 *Conventional Chin-Ups*   As many as possible up to 15 reps

20 seconds pause

3 *Cumulative Matrix Alternate Lat Machine Pulldowns:*   1 full rep, 1 half-up, 1 half-down, 2 full reps, 2 half-up, 2 half-down, 3 full reps, 3 half-up, 3 half-down, 4 full reps, 4 half-up, 4 half-down, 5 full reps

Finish

Stage VI

Sequence A

1 *Cumulative iso-Matrix Lat Machine Pulldowns:*   1 full rep, 1 rep half-up (hold for 1 second), 2 reps half-up (hold for 2 seconds), 3 reps half-up (hold for 3 seconds), 4 reps half-up (hold for 4 seconds), 5 full reps, 1 rep half-down (hold for 1 second), 2 reps half-down (hold for 2 seconds), 3 reps half-down (hold for 3 seconds), 4 reps half-down (hold for 4 seconds), 5 full reps

10 seconds pause

2 *Conventional Stiff-Legged Deadlifts:*   12–15 full reps

20 seconds pause

3 *Cumulative Matrix Alternate Lat Machine Pulldowns:*   1 full rep, 1 half-up, 1 half-down, 2 full reps, 2 half-up, 2 half-down, 3 full reps, 3 half-up, 3 half-down, 4 full reps, 4 half-up, 4 half-down, 5 full reps

10 seconds pause

4 *Conventional Stiff-Legged Deadlifts:*   12–15 full reps

Two minutes pause

Sequence B

1 *Cumulative iso-Matrix Bent-Over Rows:* 1 full rep, 1 rep half-up (hold for 1 second), 2 reps half-up (hold for 2 seconds), 3 reps half-up (hold for 3 seconds), 4 reps half-up (hold for 4 seconds), 5 full reps, 1 rep half-down (hold for 1 second), 2 reps half-down (hold for 2 seconds), 3 reps half-down (hold for 3 seconds), 4 reps half-down (hold for 4 seconds), 5 full reps

10 seconds pause

2 *Conventional Bent-Arm Pullovers;* 12–15 full reps

20 seconds pause

3 *Cumulative Matrix Alternate Bent-Over Rows:* 1 full rep, 1 half-up, 1 half-down, 2 full reps, 2 half-up, 2 half-down, 3 full reps, 3 half-up, 3 half-down, 4 full reps, 4 half-up, 4 half-down, 5 full reps

10 seconds pause

4 *Stiff-Legged Deadlifts:* 12–15 full reps

Three minutes pause

Sequence C

1 *Cumulative iso-Matrix Lat Machine Pulldowns:* 1 full rep, 1 rep half-up (hold for 1 second), 2 reps half-up (hold for 2 seconds), 3 reps half-up (hold for 3 seconds), 4 reps half-up (hold for 4 seconds), 5 full reps, 1 rep half-down (hold for 1 second), 2 reps half-down (hold for 2 seconds), 3 reps half-down (hold for 3 seconds), 4 reps half-down (hold for 4 seconds), 5 full reps

10 seconds pause

2 *Conventional Chin-Ups:* As many as possible up to 15 reps

20 seconds pause

3 *Cumulative Matrix Alternate Bent-over Rows:* 1 full rep, 1 half-up, 1 half-down, 2 full reps, 2 half-up, 2 half-down, 3 full reps, 3 half-up, 3 half-down, 4 full reps, 4 half-up, 4 half-down, 5 full reps

40 seconds pause

4 *Conventional Chin-Ups:* As many as possible up to 15 reps

Finish

Stage VII

Sequence A

1 *Matrix Alternate Lat Machine Pulldowns:* 5 full reps, 1 half-up, 1 half-down, 1 full rep, 1 half-up, 1 half-down, 2 full reps, 1 half-up, 1 half-down, 3 full reps, 1 half-up, 1 half-down, 4 full reps, 1 half-up, 1 half-down, 5 full reps

20 seconds pause

2   *Conventional iso-Matrix Lat Machine Pulldowns:*   5 full reps, 5 half-up (hold for 5 seconds), 5 half-down (hold for 5 seconds), 5 full reps

30 seconds pause

3   *Cumulative Matrix Ladder Lat Machine Pulldowns:*   1 full rep, 1 rep 1/5-up, 2 reps 2/5-up, 3 reps 3/5-up, 4 reps 4/5-up, 5 full reps, 1 rep 1/5-down, 2 reps 2/5-down, 3 reps 3/5-down, 4 reps 4/5-down, 5 full reps

40 seconds pause

4   *Mixed iso-Matrix Lat Machine Pulldowns:*   5 full reps, 3 reps half-up (hold for 3 seconds), 3 reps half-down (no holding), 3 reps half-up (no holding), 3 reps half-down (hold for 3 seconds), 5 full reps

Three minutes pause

Sequence B

1   *Matrix Alternate Bent-Over Rows:*   5 full reps, 1 half-up, 1 half-down, 1 full rep, 1 half-up, 1 half-down, 2 full reps, 1 half-up, 1 half-down, 3 full reps, 1 half-up, 1 half-down, 4 full reps, 1 half-up, 1 half-down, 5 full reps

20 seconds pause

2   *Conventional iso-Matrix Bent-Over Rows:*   5 full reps, 5 half-up (hold for 5 seconds), 5 half-down (hold for 5 seconds), 5 full reps

40 seconds pause

3   *Cumulative Matrix Ladder Bent-Over Rows:*   1 full rep, 1 rep 1/5-up, 2 reps 2/5-up, 3 reps 3/5-up, 4 reps 4/5-up, 5 full reps, 1 rep 1/5-down, 2 reps 2/5-down, 3 reps 3/5-down, 4 reps 4/5-down, 5 full reps

60 seconds pause

4   *Mixed iso-Matrix Bent-Over Rows:*   5 full reps, 3 reps half-up (hold for 3 seconds), 3 reps half-down (no holding), 3 reps half-up (no holding), 3 reps half-down (hold for 3 seconds), 5 full reps

Three minutes pause

Sequence C

1   *Conventional Bent-Arm Pullovers:*   12–15 full reps

20 seconds pause

2   *Conventional Stiff-Legged Deadlifts:*   12–15 full reps

40 seconds pause

3   *Conventional Chin-Ups:*   As many as possible up to 15 reps

Finish

Abdominal Matrix

Exercises used:

1 *Incline board sit-ups*   Lie on the incline board with knees bent and feet secured under the pad or strap. With hands on hips or chest, or extended in front of you (or held behind the head to shift the centre of gravity and make the exercise harder), bring the chin as close to the knees as possible. Lower yourself slowly to near the starting position, but without letting the back touch the board.

2 *Incline board leg raises*   Lie on your back on the incline board, head nearest the wall rack. Reach back and grasp the rack or the top of the board. Slowly raise the legs as high as possible then lower them again, keeping them straight throughout the movement. Try not to let the feet touch the board at the end of the lowering movement.

3 *Vertical bench (high chair) leg raises*   Holding the body steady on the high chair, bring the legs up as high as possible and slowly lower them again. This exercise can be performed with knees bent (the lower leg remaining perpendicular to the floor) or with legs kept straight.

4 *Crunches*   On a crunch board, or lying on the floor with knees bent and feet firmly against the wall, place the hands behind the head and raise the head and shoulders slightly, curling the spine and contracting the abs so as to crunch the upper and lower body together.

5 *Seated side twists*   Sit at the end of a bench with feet flat on the floor. Holding a bar or broomstick across the back of the shoulders, twist the shoulders as far as possible in one direction then the other, trying to feel the tensing of the obliques.

Abdominal Matrix Schedule

Stage I

Sequence A

1 *Conventional Sit-Ups:*   12–15 full reps

                30 seconds pause

2 *Matrix Leg Raises:*   5 full reps, 5 half-up, 5 half-down, 5 full reps

                50 seconds pause

3 *Conventional Abdominal Crunches:*   12–15 full reps

                Pause three minutes

Incline Board Sit-Ups

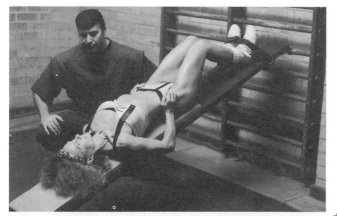

down

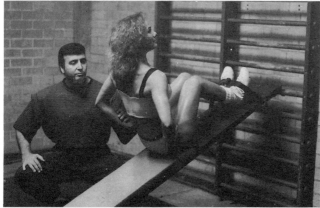

half-up

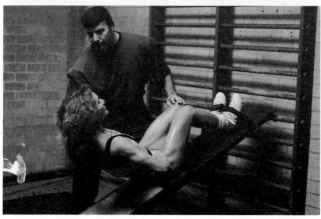

half-down

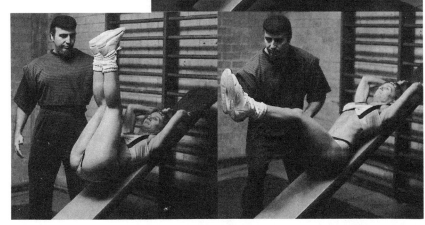

Incline Board
Leg Raises
right: down
below: up
below right: half-down

Sequence B

1 *Conventional Leg Raises:* 12–15 full reps

    30 seconds pause

2 *Matrix Sit-Ups:* 5 full reps, 5 half-up, 5 half-down, 5 full reps

    50 seconds pause

3 *Conventional Abdominal Crunches:* 12–15 full reps

    Pause three minutes

Sequence C

1 *Conventional Sit-Ups:* 12–15 full reps

    30 seconds pause

2 *Matrix Abdominal Crunches:* 5 full reps, 5 half-up, 5 half-down, 5 full reps

    50 seconds pause

3 *Conventional Leg Raises:* 12–15 full reps

    Finish

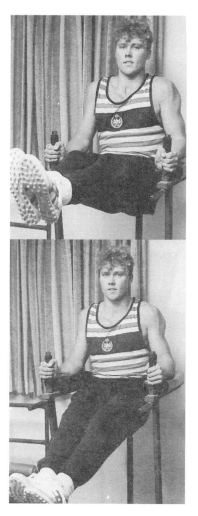

High Chair Leg Raises
straight leg
right: up
below right: half-up
below left: half-down

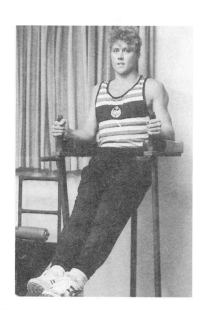

Stage II

Sequence A

1 *Matrix Sit-Ups:* 5 full reps, 5 half-up, 5 half-down, 5 full reps
                     30 seconds pause

2 *Conventional Seated Twisting:* 20 reps
                     30 seconds pause

3 *Matrix Alternate Leg Raises:* 5 full reps, 1 half-up, 1 half-down, 1
full rep, 1 half-up, 1 half-down, 2 full reps, 1 half-up, 1 half-down,
3 full reps, 1 half-up, 1 half-down, 4 full reps, 1 half-up, 1 half-down,
5 full reps

Pause three minutes

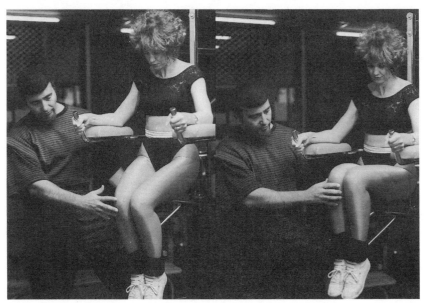

High Chair Leg Raises, bent knee   half-down   up

Sequence B

1 *Matrix Alternate Sit-Ups:*   5 full reps, 1 half-up, 1 half-down, 1 full rep, 1 half-up, 1 half-down, 2 full reps, 1 half-up, 1 half-down, 3 full reps, 1 half-up, 1 half-down, 4 full reps, 1 half-up, 1 half-down, 5 full reps

30 seconds pause

2 *Conventional Seated Twisting:*   20 reps

30 seconds pause

3 *Matrix Leg Raises:*   5 full reps, 5 half-up, 5 half-down, 5 full reps

Pause three minutes

Sequence C

1 *Matrix Sit-Ups:*   5 full reps, 5 half-up, 5 half-down, 5 full reps

30 seconds pause

2 *Conventional Seated Twisting:*   20 reps

30 seconds pause

3 *Matrix Alternate Sit-Ups:*   5 full reps, 1 half-up, 1 half-down, 1 full rep, 1 half-up, 1 half-down, 2 full reps, 1 half-up, 1 half-down, 3 full reps, 1 half-up, 1 half-down, 4 full reps, 1 half-up, 1 half-down, 5 full reps

Finish

Crunches

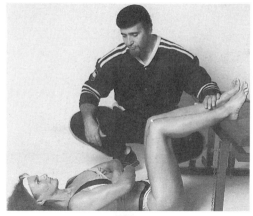

down

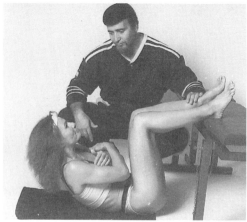

up

Stage III

Sequence A

1   *Cumulative Matrix Alternate Sit-Ups:*   1 full rep, 1 half-up, 1 half-down, 2 full reps, 2 half-up, 2 half-down, 3 full reps, 3 half-up, 3 half-down, 4 full reps, 4 half-up, 4 half-down, 5 full reps

30 seconds pause

2   *Conventional Abdominal Crunches:*   12–15 reps

50 seconds pause

3   *Matrix Alternate Leg Raises:*   5 full reps, 1 half-up, 1 half-down, 1 full rep, 1 half-up, 1 half-down, 2 full reps, 1 half-up, 1 half-down, 3 full reps, 1 half-up, 1 half-down, 4 full reps, 1 half-up, 1 half-down, 5 full reps

Pause three minutes

Sequence B

1 *Cumulative Matrix Alternate Leg Raises:* 1 full rep, 1 half-up, 1 half-down, 2 full reps, 2 half-up, 2 half-down, 3 full reps, 3 half-up, 3 half-down, 4 full reps, 4 half-up, 4 half-down, 5 full reps

30 seconds pause

2 *Conventional Abdominal Crunches:* 12–15 reps

60 seconds pause

3 *Matrix Alternate Sit-Ups:* 5 full reps, 1 half-up, 1 half-down, 1 full rep, 1 half-up, 1 half-down, 2 full reps, 1 half-up, 1 half-down, 3 full reps, 1 half-up, 1 half-down, 4 full reps, 1 half-up, 1 half-down, 5 full reps

Pause three minutes

Sequence C

1 *Cumulative Matrix Alternate Sit-Ups:* 1 full rep, 1 half-up, 1 half-down, 2 full reps, 2 half-up, 2 half-down, 3 full reps, 3 half-up, 3 half-down, 4 full reps, 4 half-up, 4 half-down, 5 full reps

30 seconds pause

2 *Conventional Abdominal Crunches:* 12–15 reps

60 seconds pause

3 *Matrix Alternate Leg Raises:* 5 full reps, 1 half-up, 1 half-down, 1 full rep, 1 half-up, 1 half-down, 2 full reps, 1 half-up, 1 half-down, 3 full reps, 1 half-up, 1 half-down, 4 full reps, 1 half-up, 1 half-down, 5 full reps

Finish

Stage IV

Sequence A

1 *Ascending Matrix Sit-Ups:* 4 full reps, 5 half-up, 6 half-down, 7 full reps

30 seconds pause

2 *Conventional High Chair Leg Raises:* 10–12 reps

50 seconds pause

3 *Descending Matrix Leg Raises:* 7 full reps, 6 half-up, 5 half-down, 4 full reps

Pause three minutes

Sequence B

1   *Matrix Alternate Sit-Ups:*   5 full reps, 1 half-up, 1 half-down, 1 full rep, 1 half-up, 1 half-down, 2 full reps, 1 half-up, 1 half-down, 3 full reps, 1 half-up, 1 half-down, 4 full reps, 1 half-up, 1 half-down, 5 full reps

30 seconds pause

2   *Conventional Seated Twisting:*   12–15 reps

50 seconds pause

3   *Ascending Matrix Leg Raises:*   4 full reps, 5 half-up, 6 half-down, 7 full reps

Pause three minutes

Sequence C

1   *Cumulative Matrix High Chair Leg Raises:*   1 full rep, 1 half-up, 1 half-down, 2 full reps, 2 half-up, 2 half-down, 3 full reps, 3 half-up, 3 half-down, 4 full reps, 4 half-up, 4 half-down, 5 full reps

30 seconds pause

2   *Conventional Seated Twisting:*   20 reps

30 seconds pause

3   *Cumulative Matrix Sit-Ups:*   1 full rep, 1 half-up, 1 half-down, 2 full reps, 2 half-up, 2 half-down, 3 full reps, 3 half-up, 3 half-down, 4 full reps, 4 half-up, 4 half-down, 5 full reps

Finish

Stage V

Sequence A

1   *Matrix Ladder Sit-Ups:*   5 full reps, 1 rep ⅕-up, 1 rep ⅖-up, 1 rep ⅗-up, 1 rep ⅘-up, 1 full rep, 1 rep ⅕-down, 1 rep ⅖-down, 1 rep ⅗-down, 1 rep ⅘-down, 1 full rep, 5 full reps

30 seconds pause

2   *Conventional Seated Twisting:*   20 reps

30 seconds pause

3   *Ascending Matrix Leg Raises:*   4 full reps, 5 half-up, 6 half-down, 7 full reps

Pause three minutes

Sequence B

1 *Cumulative Matrix Ladder Leg Raises:* 1 full rep, 1 rep ⅕-up, 2 reps ⅖-up, 3 reps ⅗-up, 4 reps ⅘-up, 5 full reps, 1 rep ⅕-down, 2 reps ⅖-down, 3 reps ⅗-down, 4 reps ⅘-down, 5 full reps

30 seconds pause

2 *Conventional Seated Twisting:* 20 reps

30 seconds pause

3 *Ascending Matrix Sit-Ups:* 4 full reps, 5 half-up, 6 half-down, 7 full reps

Pause three minutes

Sequence C

1 *Descending Matrix Sit-Ups:* 7 full reps, 6 half-up, 5 half-down, 4 full reps

30 seconds pause

2 *Conventional Seated Twisting:* 20 reps

30 seconds pause

3 *Matrix Ladder Leg Raises:* 5 full reps, 1 rep ⅕-up, 1 rep ⅖-up, 1 rep ⅗-up, 1 rep ⅘-up, 1 full rep, 1 rep ⅕-down, 1 rep ⅖-down, 1 rep ⅗-down, 1 rep ⅘-down, 1 full rep, 5 full reps

Finish

Stage VI

Sequence A

1 *Ascending iso-Matrix Sit-Ups:* 5 full reps, 1 rep half-up (hold for 1 second), 1 rep half-up (hold for 2 seconds), 1 rep half-up (hold for 3 seconds), 1 rep half-up (hold for 4 seconds), 1 rep half-up (hold for 5 seconds), 1 full rep, 1 rep half-down (hold for 1 second), 1 rep half-down (hold for 2 seconds), 1 rep half-down (hold for 3 seconds), 1 rep half-down (hold for 4 seconds), 1 rep half-down (hold for 5 seconds), 5 full reps

30 seconds pause

2 *Conventional Abdominal Crunches:* 15–20 reps

30 seconds pause

3 *Descending iso-Matrix Leg Raises:* 5 full reps, 1 rep half-up (hold for 5 seconds), 1 rep half-up (hold for 4 seconds), 1 rep half-up (hold for 3 seconds), 1 rep half-up (hold for 2 seconds), 1 rep half-up (hold for 1 second), 1 full rep, 1 rep half-down (hold for 5 seconds), 1 rep half-down (hold for 4 seconds), 1 rep half-down (hold for 3

seconds), 1 rep half-down (hold for 2 seconds), 1 rep half-down (hold for 1 seconds), 5 full reps

Two minutes pause

Sequence B

1 *Matrix Ladder Leg Raises:* 5 full reps, 1 rep ⅕-up, 1 rep ⅖-up, 1 rep ⅗-up, 1 rep ⅘-up, 1 full rep, 1 rep ⅕-down, 1 rep ⅖-down, 1 rep ⅗-down, 1 rep ⅘-down, 1 full rep, 5 full reps

30 seconds pause

2 *Conventional Seated Twisting:* 30 reps

30 seconds pause

3 *Matrix Alternate Sit-Ups:* 5 full reps, 1 half-up, 1 half-down, 1 full rep, 1 half-up, 1 half-down, 2 full reps, 1 half-up, 1 half-down, 3 full reps, 1 half-up, 1 half-down, 4 full reps, 1 half-up, 1 half-down, 5 full reps

Two minutes pause

Sequence C

1 *Ascending iso-Matrix Sit-Ups:* 5 full reps, 1 rep half-up (hold for 1 second), 1 rep half-up (hold for 2 seconds), 1 rep half-up (hold for 3 seconds), 1 rep half-up (hold for 4 seconds), 1 rep half-up (hold for 5 seconds), 1 full rep, 1 rep half-down (hold for 1 second), 1 rep half-down (hold for 2 seconds), 1 rep half-down (hold for 3 seconds), 1 rep half-down (hold for 4 seconds), 1 rep half-down (hold for 5 seconds), 5 full reps

30 seconds pause

2 *Conventional Abdominal Crunches:* 15–20 reps

30 seconds pause

3 *Descending iso-Matrix Leg Raises:* 5 full reps, 1 rep half-up (hold for 5 seconds), 1 rep half-up (hold for 4 seconds), 1 rep half-up (hold for 3 seconds), 1 rep half-up (hold for 2 seconds), 1 rep half-up (hold for 1 second), 1 full rep, 1 rep half-down (hold for 5 seconds), 1 rep half-down (hold for 4 seconds), 1 rep half-down (hold for 3 seconds), 1 rep half-down (hold for 2 seconds), 1 rep half-down (hold for 1 second), 5 full reps

Finish

Stage VII

Sequence A

1 *Conventional iso-Matrix High Chair Leg Raises:* 5 full reps, 5 half-up (hold for 5 seconds), 5 half-down (hold for 5 seconds), 5 full reps

20 seconds pause

2 *Cumulative Matrix Alternate Abdominal Board Leg Raises:* 1 full rep, 1 half-up, 1 half-down, 2 full reps, 2 half-up, 2 half-down, 3 full reps, 3 half-up, 3 half-down, 4 full reps, 4 half-up, 4 half-down, 5 full reps

30 seconds pause

3 *Matrix Ladder High Chair Leg Raises:* 5 full reps, 1 rep ⅕-up, 1 rep ⅖-up, 1 rep ⅗-up, 1 rep ⅘-up, 1 full rep, 1 rep ⅕-down, 1 rep ⅖-down, 1 rep ⅗-down, 1 rep ⅘-down, 1 full rep, 5 full reps

Two minutes pause

Sequence B

1 *Cumulative iso-Matrix Sit-Ups:* 1 full rep, 1 rep half-up (hold for 1 second), 2 reps half-up (hold for 2 seconds), 3 reps half-up (hold for 3 seconds), 4 reps half-up (hold for 4 seconds), 5 full reps, 1 rep half-down (hold for 1 second), 2 reps half-down (hold for 2 seconds), 3 reps half-down (hold for 3 seconds), 4 reps half-down (hold for 4 seconds), 5 full reps

30 seconds pause

2 *Matrix Alternate Sit-Ups:* 5 full reps, 1 half-up, 1 half-down, 1 full rep, 1 half-up, 1 half-down, 2 full reps, 1 half-up, 1 half-down, 3 full reps, 1 half-up, 1 half-down, 4 full reps, 1 half-up, 1 half-down, 5 full reps

30 seconds pause

3 *Mixed iso-Matrix Sit-Ups:* 5 full reps, 3 reps half-up (hold for 3 seconds), 3 reps half-down (no holding), 3 reps half-up (no holding), 3 reps half-down (hold for 3 seconds), 5 full reps

Two minutes pause

Sequence C

1 *Conventional iso-Matrix High Chair Leg Raises:* 5 full reps, 5 half-up (hold for 5 seconds), 5 half-down (hold for 5 seconds), 5 full reps

30 seconds pause

2 *Cumulative Matrix Alternate Sit-Ups:* 1 full rep, 1 half-up, 1 half-down, 2 full reps, 2 half-up, 2 half-down, 3 full reps, 3 half-up, 3 half-down, 4 full reps, 4 half-up, 4 half-down, 5 full reps

30 seconds pause

3 *Mixed iso-Matrix High Chair Leg Raises:* 5 full reps, 3 reps half-up (hold for 3 seconds), 3 reps half-down (no holding), 3 reps half-up (no holding), 3 reps half-down (hold for 3 seconds), 5 full reps

Finish

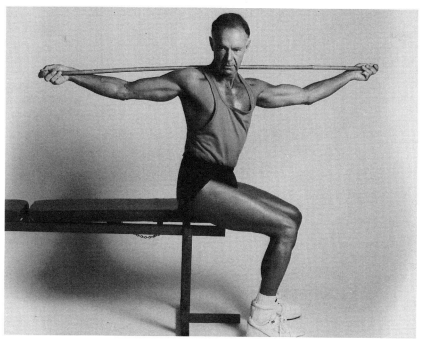

Seated Side Twists

Appendix
Muscle Charts

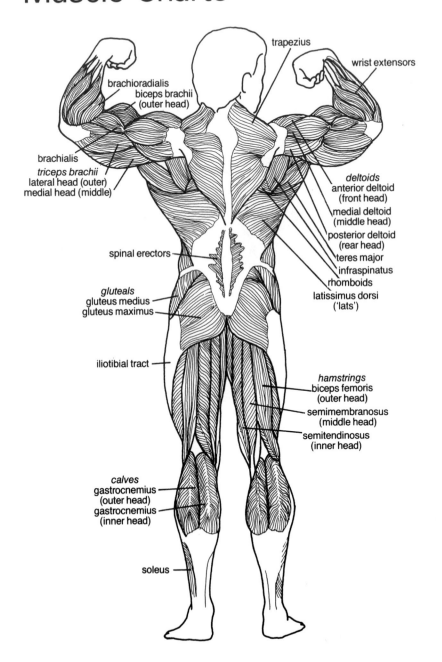

trapezius

wrist extensors

brachioradialis
biceps brachii
(outer head)

brachialis
triceps brachii
lateral head (outer)
medial head (middle)

deltoids
anterior deltoid
(front head)
medial deltoid
(middle head)
posterior deltoid
(rear head)
teres major
infraspinatus
rhomboids
latissimus dorsi
('lats')

spinal erectors

gluteals
gluteus medius
gluteus maximus

iliotibial tract

hamstrings
biceps femoris
(outer head)
semimembranosus
(middle head)
semitendinosus
(inner head)

calves
gastrocnemius
(outer head)
gastrocnemius
(inner head)

soleus

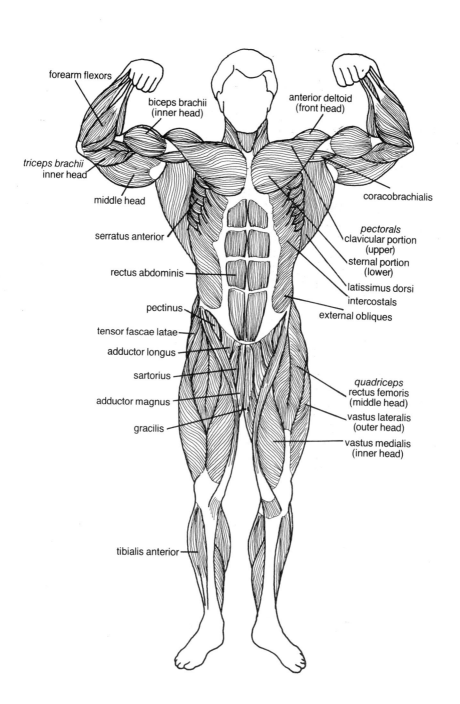

forearm flexors

biceps brachii
(inner head)

anterior deltoid
(front head)

triceps brachii
inner head

coracobrachialis

middle head

pectorals
clavicular portion
(upper)

serratus anterior

sternal portion
(lower)

latissimus dorsi

rectus abdominis

intercostals

external obliques

pectinus

tensor fascae latae

adductor longus

sartorius

quadriceps
rectus femoris
(middle head)

adductor magnus

vastus lateralis
(outer head)

gracilis

vastus medialis
(inner head)

tibialis anterior

MUSCLES OF THE NECK AND SHOULDERS

NAME	DESCRIPTION	FUNCTION	Exercises
NECK MUSCLES **MEANINGS** *Sternomastoid:* linking sternum (breastbone) with mastoid process of temporal bone; *Splenius:* Greek *splenium:* bandage *Semispinalis:* close to spine *Capitis:* muscle of the head	These include the sternomastoid, splenius and semispinalis capitis. They run either from the back and sides of the skull to the sternum or the vertebrae, or between the cervical and thoracic vertebrae. A number of them are hidden by the trapezius.	To allow the head to move relative to the body.	Shoulder shrugs neck extensions and flexions neck side-bends
DELTOID **MEANING** Shaped like triangular Greek letter *delta*	A three-headed muscle, broadly triangular in shape, which links the scapula (shoulder-blades) and clavicle (collar-bone) to the humerus (bone of the upper arm)	*Anterior* (front) head: to lift the arm to the front and assist in overhead movement; *Medial* or *lateral* (side) head: to lift the arm to the side; *Posterior* (rear) head: to draw the arm up and to the rear	Anterior head—front dumbbell raises (standing or seated) military presses (overhead barbell presses) incline presses and flyes Medial head—lateral flyes Posterior head—bent-over flyes (standing or seated) face-down incline flyes (to rear) bent-over barbell rows lying side arm raises (angled to rear)

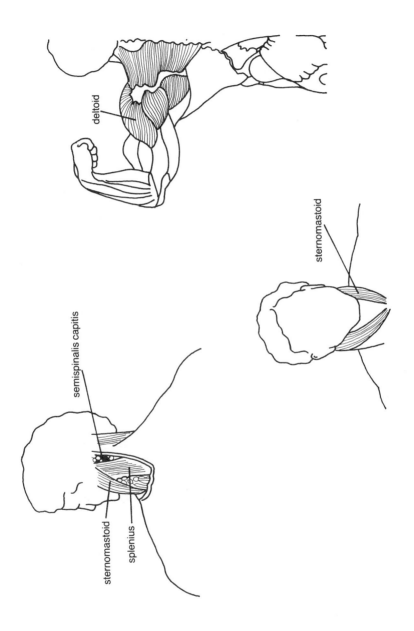

MUSCLES OF THE UPPER BACK

NAME	DESCRIPTION	FUNCTION	Exercises
TRAPEZIUS **MEANING** Trapeze-shaped.	The large, diamond-shaped sheet of muscle in the upper and middle back. It extends from the base of the skull, neck ligaments and vertebrae, and inserts on the clavicle (collar-bone) and scapula (shoulder-blades).	Ties together neck, deltoids and latissimus dorsi. Works in opposition to pulldown function of lats. Raises the shoulder-girdle, draws the shoulder-blades up, down and to the sides. Helps draw the head backward and to the sides.	dumbbell and barbell shrugs lateral flyes (dumbbell and cable) upright rows deadlifts T-bar and cable rows
TERES MAJOR **MEANING** Larger (*major*) of two muscles with rounded outline *teres*: Latin, rounded.	The outermost muscle of the upper back. It originates on the back of the scapula (shoulder-blades) and inserts on the humerus (bone of the upper arm).	Pulls the arm down and backward, rotates the arm outward.	narrow-grip pulldowns on lat machine
RHOMBOIDS and INFRASPINATUS **MEANING** *Rhomboid*: lozenge-shaped, *rhombos*: Greek, lozenge; *Infraspinatus*: situated below (*infra*) the 'spine' or ridge of the scapula (shoulder-blade).	Muscles of the upper back, lying between the teres major and trapezius. The rhomboid extends from the cervical and thoracic vertebrae, under the trapezius, to the scapula. The infraspinatus is one of a number of muscles linking the scapula to the humerus.	*Rhomboids*: to pull the shoulder-blades up and inward; *Infraspinatus*: to assist in rotating the upper arm outward.	lat pulldowns bent-over flyes

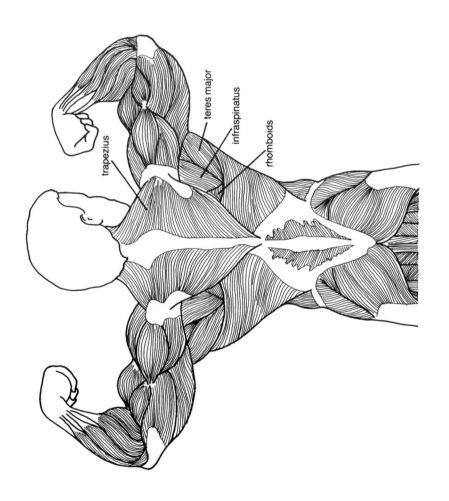

trapezius

teres major

infraspinatus

rhomboids

MUSCLES OF THE CHEST

NAME	DESCRIPTION	FUNCTION	Exercises
PECTORALIS MAJOR	The pectorals are divided into two broad bands of muscle: the upper (or *clavicular*) portion and lower (or *sternal*) portion. The upper pectoral makes up between a quarter and a third of the mass of the 'pecs': it runs from the inner border of the clavicle (collarbone) to the humerus (upper arm bone) just above the attachment of the deltoid. The lower pectoral originates along the sternum (breastbone) and the cartilage of the upper ribs.	To draw the shoulders and arms forward and inward.	flat bench presses (barbell and dumbbell)
MEANING Larger (*major*) part of the chest; *pectus:* Latin, chest.			flat bench dumbbell flyes
			Upper pectoral—
			incline presses (barbell and dumbbell, or Smith machine)
			incline flyes
			Lower pectoral—
			decline presses (barbell and dumbbell)
			decline flyes
			cable flyes
			dips
	(NB The pectoralis minor lies under the outer part of the pectoralis major, and is not visible from the surface.)		Inner pectoral—
			cable crossovers (standing or on flat bench)
			narrow-grip bench presses
			machine ('pec deck') flyes
			Outer pectoral—
			dumbbell flyes (full stretch)
			dips
			wide-grip incline presses

NAME	DESCRIPTION:	FUNCTION	Exercises
SERRATUS and INTERCOSTALS	The serratus lies on the outside of the ribs at the side of the thorax. It runs from the outer surface of the upper ribs to its insertion on the scapula (shoulder-blades). The intercostals are the muscles between the ribs.	The serratus draws the upper body closer to the legs in a crunch movement. The intercostals draw the ribs closer together.	narrow-grip pulldowns barbell and dumbbell pullovers, machine pullovers rope pulls one-arm cable pulls twisting sit-ups (intercostals)
MEANING *Serratus:* serrated, notched, *serra:* Latin, a saw; *Intercostal:* between the ribs, *costa:* Latin, rib.			

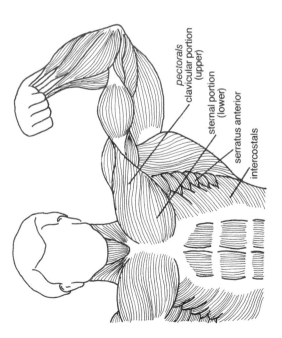

pectorals
clavicular portion (upper)

sternal portion (lower)

serratus anterior

intercostals

MUSCLES OF THE ARMS

NAME	DESCRIPTION	FUNCTION	Exercises
BICEPS BRACHII **MEANING** *Biceps*: Latin, two heads; *brachii*: Latin, of the arm	**DESCRIPTION** The two-headed muscle at the front of the upper arm. Each head is separately attached to the scapula (shoulder-blades) below the deltoid; the two heads blend into a common muscle that inserts into the radius (one of the forearm bones) below the elbow.	**FUNCTION** To flex or curl the arm; to supinate (twist upward) the forearm	**Exercises** standing barbell curls seated dumbbell curls hammer curls cheat curls incline curls concentration curls preacher curls (with barbell, dumbbells or cable machine) reverse curls lying dumbbell curls
NAME **BRACHIALIS** **MEANING** *brachium*: Latin, the arm.	**DESCRIPTION** Located next to the outer head of the biceps, between the biceps and humerus. It extends from the humerus (upper arm bone) to the ulna (one of the bones of lower arm).	**FUNCTION** To assist the biceps in certain movements.	**Exercises** reverse curls (fist downward) upright rows incline dumbbell curls
NAME **FOREARM** **EXTENSORS/FLEXORS** **MEANING** *Brachioradialis*: relating to radius bone of the arm.	**DESCRIPTION** These include principally the *brachioradialis* (the rounded muscle surface on the outer side of the lower arm) and also a number of other muscles.	**FUNCTION** To assist in pronation and supination of the lower arm and wrist. *Flexors* (inner forearm) curl the palm down and forward. *Extensors* (outer forearm): curl the knuckle back and up.	**Exercises** *Flexors:* wrist curls *Extensors:* reverse curls hammer curls reverse wrist curls incline dumbbell curls

NAME	DESCRIPTION	FUNCTION
TRICEPS BRACHII	The three-headed muscle at the rear of the upper arm. Each head originates separately at the back of the humerus (upper arm bone) or on the scapula (shoulder-blades), but the three heads go into a common tendon which inserts into the ulna (one of the forearm bones) near the elbow-joint.	All three heads (*long* or inner, *lateral* or outer and *medial* or middle) extend the forearm and assist in pronation (twisting downwards) of the wrist. The head principally exercised depends largely on the angle of the wrist.
MEANING		
Triceps: Latin, three heads.		

Exercises

standing triceps pushdowns (on lat or cable machine)
overhead triceps presses (standing or seated) with barbell or dumbbell
overhead triceps presses (standing or kneeling) on cable machine
narrow-grip bench presses
dips (on dip bar or between benches)
kickbacks
lying triceps extensions
For outer head—
hands in thumbs-up position (rope pushdowns, dips, kickbacks, behind-the-neck extensions with rope)
For inner head—
thumbs turned inward, little finger no higher than thumb (triceps pushdowns with bar, one-arm pushdowns, reverse grip pressdowns)

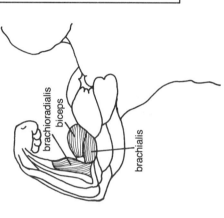

biceps brachii (inner head)

forearm flexors

triceps brachii (inner head)

brachioradialis

biceps

brachialis

MUSCLES OF THE MIDDLE AND LOWER BACK

NAME / MEANING	DESCRIPTION	FUNCTION	Exercises
NAME LATISSIMUS DORSI **MEANING** Latin, broadest part of the back.	**DESCRIPTION** The large muscle of the middle back which extends from the lumbar and lower thoracic vertebrae, sacrum, ilium and lower ribs, to its insertion on the humerus (upper arm bone).	**FUNCTION** To pull the arms and shoulders downward and backward.	**Exercises** For overall development— chin-ups (in front of neck) T-bar rows one-arm dumbbell rows machine pullovers For upper lats— wide-grip chins behind neck wide-grip lat machine pulldowns For lower lats— seated cable rows close-grip chins close or medium grip pulldowns
NAME ERECTOR SPINAE **MEANING** Latin, spinal erector.	**DESCRIPTION** A group of four separate but grouped muscles running all the way down the back from neck to sacrum. Only the lower part (from the bottom of the trapezius downward) is visible on the surface.	**FUNCTION** To support and hold the spine erect; to permit straightening back from a bent positon.	**Exercises** deadlifts 'good-mornings' back hyperextensions

NAME
GLUTEUS MAXIMUS

MEANING
The longest (*maximus*) muscle of the buttocks; *gloutos*: Greek, rump.

DESCRIPTION
A large muscle at the back of the hip, extending from the back of the sacrum, lumbar area and sides of the coccyx, to its insertion on the back of the femur (thigh-bone) and the fascia lata (side face) of the thigh.

FUNCTION
To extend the thigh and rotate it outward.

Exercises
squats
lunges (forward and sideways)
leg abduction exercises on abductor machine or cable machine

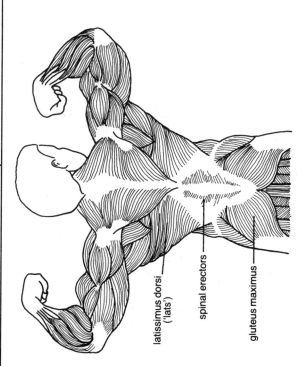

latissimus dorsi ('lats')

spinal erectors

gluteus maximus

MUSCLES OF THE ABDOMEN

NAME / MEANING	DESCRIPTION	FUNCTION	Exercises
NAME RECTUS ABDOMINIS **MEANING** Straight muscle of abdomen; *rectus*: Latin, straight.	**DESCRIPTION** The muscle which extends up and down the front of the abdominal wall. It originates on the crest of the pubis and inserts into the cartilage of the 5th, 6th and 7th ribs. The right and left sides are separated by a strip of cartilage (the linea alba).	**FUNCTION** To flex the spinal column, depress the thorax (rib-cage) and draw the chest towards the pelvis.	**Exercises** sit-ups Roman chair sit-ups knee raises (on board, flat bench or high chair) hanging knee raises (from chin bar) crunches
NAME OBLIQUES **MEANING** *obliquus*: Latin, slanting, inclined.	**DESCRIPTION** The *external obliques* run along the side of the rectus abdominis, with fibres running diagonally sideward and upward. The *internal obliques* lie lower than and inwards of the external obliques. 　The origin of the external obliques and insertion of the internal obliques is on the lower ribs.	**FUNCTION** To twist the body by rotating the pelvis on the chest and rotating the spinal column.	**Exercises** twisting sit-ups twisting knee raises on incline board and flat bench twisting knee raises (hanging from chin bar) side bends bent-over twists lying side leg raises

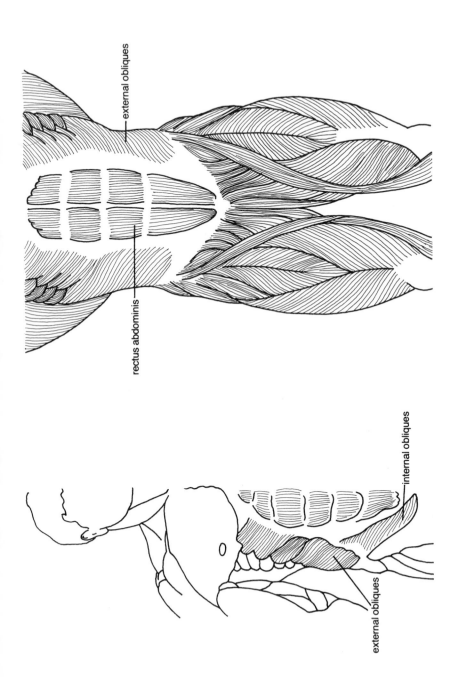

external obliques

rectus abdominis

internal obliques

external obliques

MUSCLES OF THE LEGS

NAME	DESCRIPTION	FUNCTION	Exercises
HAMSTRING GROUP, THIGH FLEXORS **MEANING** *Biceps femoris*: two-headed muscle of the thigh (Latin, *femur*). *Semimembranosus, semitendinosus*: resembling a membrane or tendon.	The muscles at the rear of the upper leg, consisting of: (a) the *biceps femoris* (leg biceps), a two-headed muscle attaching to the pelvis and the femur at the top, the tibia and fibula (bones of the lower leg) at the bottom; (b) the *semimembranosus* and *semitendinosus*, long muscles running alongside the leg biceps, from the hips to the lower leg.	To flex or 'curl' the lower leg relative to the upper, and to rotate the leg.	leg curls (lying or standing) stiff-legged deadlifts 'good-mornings'
NAME: LOWER LEG TENSORS/FLEXORS **MEANING** *gastrocnemius*: Greek, *gaster* (belly) and *kneme* (tibia); the 'belly' of the lower leg muscle *soleus*: Latin, *solea*; shaped like a sole—either the fish or the sole of the foot *tibialis anterior*: Latin, front muscle of the shin bone.	These consist of: (a) the *gastrocnemius* (or calf muscle) at the back of the lower leg, running from the lower part of the femur (thigh bone) to the heel via an Achilles tendon; (b) the *soleus*, running from the fibula and tibia (lower leg bones) to the heel and situated between the calf and the heel; (c) the *tibialis anterior*, which runs up the front of the lower leg beside the tibia (shin-bone).	**FUNCTION:** To extend and flex the foot; to assist in ankle-joint extension.	standing calf-raises donkey calf-raises calf-raises on leg-press machine seated calf-raises (to isolate soleus) stretching versions of the above (heel lower than sole of foot) to isolate tibialis

NAME	DESCRIPTION	FUNCTION	Exercises
QUADRICEPS GROUP	The muscles at the front of the upper leg, consisting of:	To extend and tense the upper leg.	squats (including front squats and hack squats)
MEANING	(a) the *rectus femoris*, the V-shaped muscle at the front of the thigh, attached to the ilium bone of the pelvis and covering the *vastus intermedius*;		leg presses
Quadriceps: Latin, four heads.			leg extensions
Rectus femoris: 'straight' part of thigh;	(b) the *vastus lateralis*, the large muscle on the outside of the thigh, attached to the length of the femur (thigh-bone);		
femur: Latin, thigh;			
vastus: Latin, huge.	(c) the *vastus medialis*, the muscle of the inner thigh, slightly lower than the lateralis, attached to the inner side of the femur.		

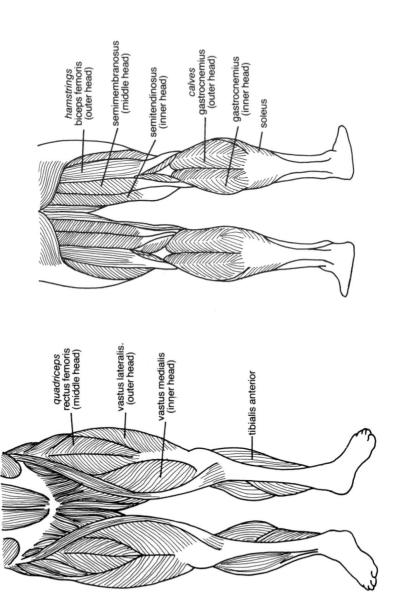

quadriceps
rectus femoris
(middle head)

vastus lateralis.
(outer head)

vastus medialis
(inner head)

tibialis anterior

hamstrings
biceps femoris
(outer head)

semimembranosus
(middle head)

semitendinosus
(inner head)

calves
gastrocnemius
(outer head)

gastrocnemius
(inner head)

soleus

- Matrix – each part – 2x per wk.

- Schedule – 6/7 days,
    1-2 days aerob
    0-1 days rest
    Matrix 1 U & 1 L part

- 3-4 sec. U , 2 sec D (neg) "Slow" reps

- Weight Reduct – no Abs 1st 7 wks
                Leg
                Chest   ★ 'est muscle groups
                Should

- Eat – Water Fiber 6 meals Protein load (70)

CHEST	Bench Press	TRICEP	Lying Press
	Inc/Dec Press		Stand Press
	Dumbbell/Inc. Fly		Tri Pushdn
	Pushups		Dip
	Bfx Fly	DELTOID	Roll Press
	Dip.		Block Side Laterals
THIGH	Squat		Press Behind Neck
	Leg Press		Press W/o neck
	Leg Curl		Block Front Raises
	Leg Ext.		Upright Row
BICEP	Curl togeth		
	Curl sep		